Going-Natural
How to fall in love with nappy hair

Mireille Liong-A-Kong

Foreword by Patricia Gaines a.k.a. Deecoily,
Founder of nappturality.com

D0803066

Published by Sabi Wiri Inc. ®

Published by Sabi Wiri Inc.
Brooklyn, NY

Cover design: Mireille Liong-A-Kong

Dedication

For the greatest parents in the world,
Hertha Liong-A-Kong-Ritfeld
and Daisy Liong-A-Kong,
who were always there for me.

Acknowledgements

Patricia Gains a.k.a. Dee: Thank you so much for writing the foreword. You are the best, a great inspiration for all women of color.

Sharine Dawn: Thank you for taking the time to read and edit in my hour of desperation.

Dr. JoAnne Cornwell: Thanks for explaining the Sisterlocks concept to me.

All the models who sent and allowed me to use their pictures: Dolores, Jenteel, Satcha, Sharyn, Sandy, Nicole, Roshini, Fatima, Sherize, Rachelle, Kaissa, Satcha, Mamke, Roline, JoAnne, Deidre Small, Deej, SweetAfrica, Myrena Sint Jago, Richelle Braithwaite a.k.a. Riqui, Porche , Terza, Saskia Norine Abena and Graciella: Thank you so very much.

All the visitors of kroeshaar.com and my supportive audience in Holland and Suriname: You are the ones who got me started: "Dank je wel" and "Grantangi".

All the visitors of nappturality.com: Your advice, hints and tips are truly motivating. Please continue to offer your thoughts.

My husband and the rest of my family: Thank you for your patience.

Foreword

By Patricia Gaines a.k.a. "Deecoily"
Founder of nappturality.com

If, five years ago, someone had come up to me and said "You'll be writing the foreword for a book on Black women's natural hair," I'd have looked at them like they were crazy. "Natural hair? You must be kidding," I would say. "Why in the WORLD would I wear my hair looking like THAT?"

I knew nothing about my natural hair. It was that mess that grew out of my head. Those ugly, unmanageable, dry, kinky, coily, wavy, bendy strands I couldn't comb that gave me such grief -- which was only relieved by using scalp-burning chemicals and hair-singeing heat. It was that unprofessional, bad, embarrassing stuff that if I were to wear in public, would doom me to everlasting singledom and job failure because, surely, no employer would employ me nor would a suitable life partner love me with hair like... "THAT." So I would beat it, pull it, break it into submission until it was STRAIGHT!

How many of us can remember that defining incident when we decided our hair was unacceptable in its natural state? Was it something someone said? Was it a painful combing session or a scalp-torturing rubber band removal? I don't think it matters much. The important thing is, we are coming full circle and regaining what we lost... our whole selves.

Well, here I am; five years and a lifetime later, full of NAPPtural hair and pride. I wear my hair in the state it was intended to be worn, and I have never felt freer. These feelings of joy and sky-high self-esteem that go along with the wearing of your hair NAPPturally is something born again naturals feel the need to share. Such elation and freedom after years of torture, hiding, shame and pain drive the desire to talk and meet with others who share the experience. We also want to reach out and touch those who may be thinking about or curious about... the resurgence of the pride in wearing of NAPPtural hair.

Books like this one serve a wonderful purpose. They tell us we are not alone - that this soul-freeing experience is one that is also felt by other Black women who for years have oppressed their hair and their minds into believing there was something "wrong" with them. That the way they were created was less than perfect.

The pain, the scarring, the hair breakage and the inevitable hair loss must stop. We, and our daughters, will only benefit with the healthy knowledge we pass on to them about every part of their bodies while in the process instilling them with pride in themselves. Their skin, their features and their hair are all beautiful in their own right. Black women need to celebrate their beauty, and this book is a great place to start.

I commend Mireille and you, the reader, for reaching out and absorbing this knowledge.

~Dee~

Author's note

My journey, my motivation

Like so many nappy-haired girls, I started to relax my hair when I was 14. At that age, looking mature was very important. Since I had been wearing an afro from age eight, a change of style was extra welcome. Needless to say, I loved my new look and enjoyed my grown-up straight hair. The joy did not last for long. Dancing to only one song at a very anticipated teenage party would make my carefully styled hair collapse. The humidity and sweat made me look like a drowned cat. Because participation in different kinds of sports was also part of my teenage life, my hair was difficult to keep in place and my straightened tresses became a constant source of concern. Since I didn't know what else to do with my hair, I just tried to learn to live with it. Sometimes my hair was a real mess, but most of the time I managed. The chemical treatment was something I felt reluctant to each and every time and I certainly did not like the high maintenance, but I resigned myself to the whole process and I coped.

After college, my hair really became more than a constant source of concern; it became a burden. Maybe it was the change of environment, from a tropical one to one with four seasons, but suddenly I had to deal with severe breakage. My hair was also thin, lifeless and dry. Out of desperation, I started to wear braids with extensions. It was uncomfortable in the beginning. I had to get used to the fake, long braids but felt that it would be temporary anyway. I only needed to grow my hair back so I could relax it again and take much better care of it. I was sure that that would solve all the problems. Needless to say, this didn't work. I went from one expensive professional hairdresser to the next, from a three month to an eight week touchup-period, from a regular lye to a mild, no-lye relaxer and vice versa, but nothing could stop my hair from breaking once it was chemically processed. I was caught in a vicious cycle of braiding my hair, growing lovely healthy naps, then relaxing again only to have my kinks break down to my scalp again.

One day while this nearly bald spot was sadly gazing at me in the mirror, I asked myself, "Why am I doing this?" Why do I keep straightening my hair so compulsively? It is no fun having your scalp burned every couple of weeks, the maintenance is certainly not easy nor cheap and on top of that, my healthy naps were clearly deteriorating after flourishing while wearing braids. It was at that point that I decided, "No more." I had no clue what I would or could do with my nappy hair but my mind was made up, no more straightening.

The positive aspect about the vicious cycle was that I had become an expert in caring for extensions and taking them out. So, although I couldn't even make a decent braid, I didn't have any "hair-aches" for a year. My natural naps were flourishing and I wasn't really concerned about the next step of learning how to style my natural hair until I had to. After taking out my extensions, washing my hair, combing it and making my usual funny looking braids, I routinely put on my hat and went on my way to the steady braider I had known now for more than one year. This was on a Sunday and I must have rung her bell a dozen times because I just couldn't believe that she wasn't there. I was stunned and freaked out! The next day would be a working day and I had no clue what to do with my full head of healthy naps. One thing was sure; as funny as those braids were to me, wearing them to work didn't seem amusing at all, and showing up with a hat at the job was no option either. Dependent as I was on the mercy of the home braiders, I called every number from possible braiders but no luck. Of course there were plenty of Black hair salons around that loved to take kinks out with a perm. Since I couldn't style my naps and I was out of braiders, I had little choice and ended up in a salon chair for a relaxer. With a mixed feeling of rage, sadness and despair, I felt the relaxer burning my scalp taking out the kinks of my poor healthy naps once again. My nearly bald spot was gone and I knew it would be back not long after the treatment. But who was to blame? The braider who stood me up, the hairdresser who simply did her job or the relaxer itself that was too harsh for my hair? Sure, I could blame everything and everyone but wasn't it my choice to sit there because I couldn't style my own naps?

Ultimately, this desperate act turned into a moment of truth. Blaming the rest of the world and feeling sorry for my naps was not going to improve my hair's health. Besides that, it troubled me that I couldn't take care of my own hair just because it was natural. This was when I realized that I needed to learn at least the basics about styling natural Afrikan hair. It couldn't be that difficult and there had to be more acceptable hairstyles other than an afro or extension braids. In my eagerness to learn, I started to search for literature to help me solve the kinky mysteries. Since there were no local books about the subject, I ordered every book available via the Internet and collected the few Black hair magazines the stores offered. Unconsciously this is where my natural journey really started and it has been a wonderful experience ever since.

This time, I was consciously going natural and started with easy styles like tucked in braids. A braider would still do my hair initially, but every few weeks, I would redo the style myself. Inspired by the magazines, I tried Twists and Bantus. Before I knew it, I had the hang of basic natural hair care. This was unbelievable because I considered myself left-handed before. My hair grew like weeds and nothing could beat the feeling of touching my lively, healthy, flourishing naps. Not even people who didn't like my nappy hair could take away this sensation. My naps made me feel like Samson - invincible. I realized the power of hair and since then I developed a special kind of love for my natural naps.

It is this feeling that I would like to share with every woman of color who ever had trouble caring for her natural hair. I only hope this book passes on a little of my affection for nappy hair because our naps have been undervalued far too much for far too long.

Going Natural

Going natural is a remarkable, astounding journey. After presuming that kinky hair is bad and unsuitable for centuries, learning to truly appreciate natural Afrikan hair is not that simple. Consequently, recognizing that you *can* look good wearing natural hair may take some time. Learning to deal with your tresses naturally is another challenge you'll have to face because, after decades of straightening, most of us have forgotten what our own texture is like, let alone how to groom or style natural hair.

Still, going natural is not as difficult as it may seem. First, we have to forget nearly all that we have learned about hair care. Most of what we have learned about hairstyling is based on straight or straightened hair and grooming natural Afrikan hair is completely different. Secondly, we have to get familiar with our natural naps and learn how to nurture them.

With a little courage and some patience, you will find out that Afrikan hair is not hard to groom or to manage. It is just *different*. Every step of your journey will be worth the effort because the reward is priceless: soft, healthy, flourishing naps.

You have choices

Cutting your hair short is not the only way to begin your natural journey. In fact, there are a couple of other ways to start going natural and there is no single best way to do this. Every journey is a personal one and you are the best judge to decide on which option will suit you most favorably. The options to start your natural journey are:

~ *TRANSITIONING*: this means letting the natural hair grow but keeping the processed hair and gradually cutting it off. Transitioning will be discussed in Chapter 5.

~ *THE BIG CHOP*: this means cutting off all processed hair and actually starting the journey with natural hair. The Big Chop will be discussed in Chapter 6.

Either option offers two other possibilities:

~ *LOCS:* whether you decide to transition or chop you can start at anytime. Locs will be discussed in Chapter 7.

~ *EXTENSIONS:* even if your hair is as short as one inch, extensions can be used to give your hair a rest and a chance to grow, whether you did the big chop or transitioning. Extensions and weaves will be discussed in Chapter 8.

These options offer more than enough versatile styles to make everyone happy. You can look your best and you won't become bored. If you did the big chop and you want a different look, you can try extensions or an afro weave. If you are tired of trying transitioning styles, you can do the big chop or try switching to extensions. And, it doesn't matter how far you are in the process of going natural, with today's techniques you can start locing your hair when you feel ready to do so.

If you feel that you are limited in your options, due to severe hair damage such as bald spots, see a dermatologist and a professional natural hairstylist to consider your alternatives.

Remember that no matter which way you choose to start your journey, the goal is getting there: learning how to appreciate and nurture your natural hair. Either option and every style that you choose will teach you about yourself and your natural hair. Finding hairstyles that suit you and make you look your best, will help you enjoy the experience of going natural. Feeling confident and beautiful are keys to take pleasure in your journey. This, in turn, will allow you to naturally get comfortable with your kinky hair and embrace the natural you.

Collect hairstyles

Certainly, you have seen enough attractive kinky hairstyles to wonder, "Can I look good wearing my hair natural?" Sure you can! Since looking good and feeling confident are essential to enjoying your journey, Going-Natural will help you to look as attractive as the hairstyles you so admire.

Begin collecting all the natural hairstyles that you like, and use these wonderful styles as inspirations to start your journey. Magazines are a good source to collect pictures, and with a digital camera or a picture phone, you can quickly record your favorite styles. The Internet is an excellent source but ask permission before you save or print a picture.

Collect diverse styles if you like versatility, from short naturals to long box braids. The only criteria should be that the style would look appealing on you. If you aren't sure, this old trick might help: cut your face from a photo, hold it against the hairstyle picture and see if the style will suit you.

Don't limit your collection to a certain number. Collect as many styles as you can. Your favorite hairstyles will be helpful throughout the whole natural journey.

Your first natural goal

Choose one hairstyle out of your collection of favorites and make it your first natural goal. This is the first hairstyle that you want to experience with your own natural hair. Select any style you wish as long as it is completely natural and at least three inches. It will take about six months to reach this length and that's about the minimum time you'll need to learn the basics about your natural hair. Extension styles are not allowed as your first natural goal, unless you want to recreate the style with your own natural hair. Do not worry about the length or the condition of your hair right now. The journey should lead you to the desired natural hairstyle.

In the meantime

Now that your first goal is clear, you can start planning the way to get there. We will call the time you spend to get there "in the meantime." In the meantime, the path to your first natural goal should also be paved with nice hairstyles because we always want to look good and there is no reason not to. We will call the styles you wear in the meantime "in-between" hairstyles. All your collected pictures, except the one you choose for your first natural goal, could be seen as your "in-between" hairstyles. In fact, you start your journey with "in between" hairstyles.

"In the meantime" is a very important period; it is quality time for you and your hair and you will learn three major lessons. You will:

1. *Rediscover your texture*
   Many of us don't know our natural naps because for as long as we can remember, we have had our hair straightened. "In the meantime" will allow your hair to heal and your natural texture to reveal itself so that you will get the chance to know your own unique kinks.

2. *Learn how to care for your wonderful naps*
   Not only will you learn about natural Afrikan hair care, but you will also find out what works best for your hair.

3. Learn about hairstyling
Experimenting with different hairstyles will allow you to learn the fundamentals of natural hairstyling.

Timeline

Hair is continuously growing, but it will take some time before your hair has reached the desired length to experience your first natural goal. How much time will depend on the condition of your hair and scalp. If you have used chemical straighteners for years, you can be assure that your hair and scalp have been adversely affected by their use. Even if there is no visible damage, it is very likely that hair needs time to recover after chemical treatments.

Another important factor is the speed of your hair growth. Hair grows half an inch monthly on average, so if you are healthy and your hair growth is average, you should be able to realize your first natural goal within six to eight months for a short hairstyle and within 10 to 12 months if you choose one with longer hair. Use the hair growth guideline to estimate how long it will take you to reach your first natural goal.

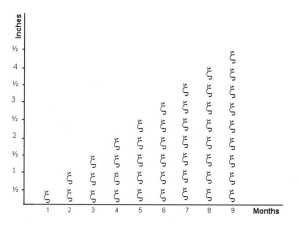

Figure 1. The hair growth guideline

(How long before you reach your first natural goal?)

Picture your journey

When you have a collection of favorite hairstyles, a natural goal and a timeframe, you can easily plan your journey. Start selecting your in-between hairstyles from your collection of favorites. Since it normally takes one to two years to grow a full head of hair, select 11 to 23 hairstyles and add a picture of yourself with your current hairstyle to make a collage. Each picture represents the hairstyle that you will wear in a certain month. Once you get the hairstyle, you replace the picture by your own photo. This way you will be able to see your hair's progress over a one to two year period. You may not need that many hairstyles if you are planning to wear the same hairstyle for more than one month. For example, braid extensions can carry over for two to three months. Just make extra copies of a hairstyle that you wish to wear for a longer time to match the number of months and the number of pictures.

Begin with a picture of yourself wearing your current hairstyle and follow by arranging your collected hairstyles in the order you want to wear them. It is easier to split up the journey in periods of six months, as it keeps things clear. See figure 2. You will have an overview of your journey in periods of half a year. So arrange your pictures in four rows of six hairstyles like in "Figure 2 Picture your journey." Schedule al least two milestones; your natural goal and the big chop. Later you can mark, color and keep notes from milestones and remarkable moments. When you are finished with the collage, you should be able to picture your journey by looking at your collage. If this gives you a happy feeling, you are ready to begin and enjoy your journey.

Your personal journal online

You can have your personal journey pictured online. The website, http://going-natural.com, was specifically designed to help women on their natural journeys. Whether you are in the process of going natural or already natural, this site will allow you to keep an online journal, select hairstyles, upload pictures and connect with other naturals. Many sisters, who have been in the exact same situation as you are now, are more than willing to answer questions and support you on your natural journey. Visit going-natural.com to join and become part of this supportive, online community.

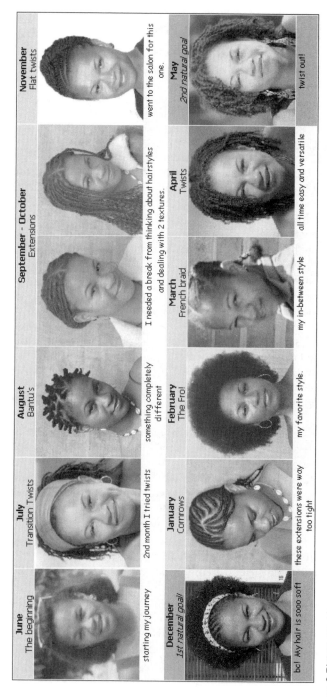

Figure 2 Picture your journey

http://going-natural.com

The truth about going natural

Unlike what most people believe, dealing with natural Afrikan hair is not a difficult task. The most difficult task is dealing with misconceptions that we have regarded as facts for so long that they became an accepted reality for many of us. In this section we'll discuss ways these misconceptions came to be and how to battle them.

Norm versus normal

Who is not familiar with the phrase "Your hair is nappy; it needs fixing?" This means that it's time for a touchup and implies that pure Afrikan hair is undesirable. The worst aspect is that our hair care routines - and in many cases even our lives - are based upon and revolve around these kinds of notions. The beliefs are so profound that, of course, it will take some time before people will be able to let these misconceptions go.

These routines and beliefs about our hair did not just appear out of the blue one day. A closer look will tell you that our routines - the way we comb, wash and style our hair - are merely based on a straight hair care model. This is hardly a surprise. Straight hair has been a dominating beauty standard in our society for such a long time that it became the norm and we unconsciously adopted it as a model for all hair types. However, the standards for straight hair are not necessarily correct or healthy for kinky hair. By using these standards as a norm for all other different hair types, we confused the *norm* with what is *normal*.

This pattern has occurred for centuries throughout history. Another example that we all can relate to is the "size six norm." Even though being a size six is the prevalent beauty standard and the majority of us strive to fit this norm, we cannot confuse this "size six norm" with "normal." Beautiful women come in all sizes. Actually, most women do not fit into a size six category, so in fact, that size is not even "normal." Still, it rules as a standard and we have unconsciously adopted it as a norm for everybody.

We must clear up these contradictions. You don't need to be a size six to be beautiful. Likewise, your hair does not need to be straight to be beautiful. Beautiful hair comes in all textures and in all lengths. Additionally, Afrikan hair responds differently to routines designed for straight hair, but that does not imply that our hair is unmanageable, bad or abnormal. Normal Afrikan hair is naturally singular so it responds differently; it has other needs and that's why we need other norms and routines. However, before we get into our afro routines, let's first try to clear up some stubborn misconceptions.

Misconceptions

Afrikan hair can't grow long
It is still a pervasive belief that Afrikan hair can't grow long. When you offer a cursory look around, you hardly see women of color with long hair. This is deceiving because naturally straight hair is compared to chemically straightened hair. Hair that is chemically treated to look straight has been through numerous processes to keep it straight. Apart from the chemical process, which is already damaging, it is very likely that blow-drying and ironing are done on a regular basis to keep the hair straight. This makes the comparison unfair because naturally straight hair does not need all the unhealthy treatments to keep the strands straight.

A closer look will show that Black women with very long hair usually wear natural hairstyles like dreadlocks. To make a fair comparison, compare long, natural, straight hair to naturally cultivated dreadlocks. Try to imagine all women who are now wearing perms wearing luscious locs instead and then make the comparison again. Compare the long locs with long straight hair. Do you still believe that afro hair cannot grow long?

Natural Afrikan hair is hard to manage
The misconception that Afrikan hair is hard to manage is based on the customs of daily combing and daily styling one's hair. Natural Afrikan hair does not need combing or styling everyday because hairstyles stay unimpaired for at least one week on average. In addition, most combs are unsuitable for natural Afrikan hair. That means being able to quickly comb through the hair on a daily basis cannot be used as a standard to define our hair as "hard to manage." Defining nappy hair as unmanageable based on the above standards would be like, defining straight hair as unmanageable because it is difficult to braid straight hair and it can hardly keep a braid, a cornrow or a curl. It doesn't make sense, does it?

Straightening Afrikan hair makes hair care easier
It may seem easy to comb through and style straightened hair on a daily basis but it certainly is not easier to care for relaxed hair. If this were true, where do you suppose the majority of our hair problems come from? Why do so many women of color wear weaves and braids these days? Contrary to popular belief, relaxed hair is high, actually very high, maintenance. In fact, chemically altered hair is more difficult to care for than natural hair because

of the chemical damage to hair. Relaxers first destroy the outer layer of a hair strand and then subsequently break the hair structure so that the hair becomes straight. That is why Afrikan hair needs extra care after it has been permed. It is more vulnerable. You can read more about how relaxers work in Appendix B.

Relaxers not only make it harder to maintain healthy hair, they also limit us in our lifestyles. To maintain a straight and healthy looking hairstyle, we condition, roller set, blow-dry, wrap or tong our hair. After all efforts we put into creating a hairstyle, we do everything to keep the hairstyle and we limit ourselves to activities that will not hinder the style. We don't exercise because perspiration messes up our hair, as does swimming, and a lot of other outdoor activities. The truth is, chemicals really do not make life easier and they make it absolutely harder to maintain healthy hair.

Natural Afrikan hair is difficult to style
Styling natural hair is not difficult at all. It may take some time getting used to like when you first learned to roller set, wrap, blow-dry or hot iron your hair, but natural hair is no more difficult than that. Actually, compared to actions like blow-drying and wrapping, the basics of natural hair care are a breeze. The most difficult practice to get used to will be untangling the hair, but besides that, it comes down to twisting and braiding. The majority of us are already familiar with these basics, so it won't be difficult to learn to style your own hair.

Natural Afrikan hair offers limited hairstyling
This is far from the truth. Afrikan hair is probably the most versatile hair type there is. Styles range from casual and classic up-do's to hip and extravagant. In fact, Afrikan hair is so unique that many styles designed for our hair type are impossible to recreate with other hair types. We should embrace this uniqueness.

Natural hair care is too time-consuming compared to relaxed hair
This is just one more misconception accepted as truth without question. Let's do the math. Table 1 Table of maintenance shows a maintenance/time schedule of different hairstyles. To make a fair evaluation, we compared the maintenance of medium hair lengths for different hairstyles on a bimonthly basis.

Relaxed	Hairstyle in hours	Extensions	Twists	Cornrows
3	Touch-up - Getting hairstyle	8	4	3
-	Taking Hairstyle out	12	3	2
3	Total hours	20	7	5
3	Bi-montly HS in hours	20	14	20

Weekly	Maintenance in Minutes	Weekly	4-weekly	Bi-Weekly
20	Washing	20	20	20
45	Conditioning	-	45	45
5	Untangling	-	60	60
30	Roller-set/Blow drying	-	-	-
45	Hood dryer/Curling iron	-	-	-
145	Total minutes	20	125	125
1160	Bi-monthly in minutes	160	250	500
19.3	Bi-monthly WM in hours	2.7	4.2	8.3

	Daily maintenance in Minutes			
15	Combing - Styling	1	1	1
15	Nightly preparations	1	1	1
30	Total Minutes	2	2	2
1800	Bi-monthly total in miniutes	120	120	120
30	Bi-monthly DM in Hours	2	2	2

	Bi-Monthly haircare and mantainenance			
Relaxed		Extensions	Twists	Cornrows
3	Hairstyle	20	14	20
19	Weekly maintenance	2.7	4.2	8.3
30	Daily maintenance	2	2	2
52.3	Total hours	24.7	20.2	30.3

Table 1 Table of maintenance

* HS=Hair Styling, WM= Weekly Maintenance, DM=Daily Maintenance

Maintenance of Relaxers
Women routinely have touchups every four to eight weeks to maintain a straightened hairstyle. This process takes three hours on average at a salon. Parting the hair, basing the scalp and applying straightener will take about 30 minutes. Rinsing, neutralizing, washing and conditioning will consume another 40 minutes. Since trimming the hair is recommended after a touchup, an additional 30 minutes is included to complete this. Roller setting or blow-drying takes a minimum of 30 minutes. After this, either the hood-dryer or curling iron will take another 45 minutes.

This means that a typical person will spend at least three hours every four to eight weeks to straighten her hair. See the left column "Relaxed hair".

To maintain a relaxed hairstyle, a person spends a little more than two hours per week to wash, condition, dry and style the hair.
This means that a person will spend eight times two hours and 10 minutes - 18 hours bimonthly to maintain a straightened hairstyle.

Daily styling and nightly preparations take about less than an hour per day - about 15 minutes in the morning and 15 minutes before bedtime. This is an average because some people spend an hour doing their hair with a curling iron and some just put their hair in a ponytail in the morning. Nightly preparations don't take that long. Most women just comb and wrap the hair, which will take 10 minutes. Other women will take time to roll their hair, which takes about 30 minutes.

This means that a typical person will spend at least 30 hours every two months to care for her straightened hair.

By the end of the two months, a person with relaxed hair has spent as much as 52 hours on hair care!

Maintenance of Extensions
We chose to compare the maintenance of a relaxer to the maintenance of braided extensions because most people are aware that it time consuming to complete such hairstyles. In general, a braider would need anywhere from five to 10 hours to complete a medium size braid style depending on the skills of a braider. We chose medium-size braids because micro-braids are bad for your hair; braiding the hair into too small box braids causes hair breakage. See the chapter "Weaves and Extensions." We choose to take more than the average time. Let's say it takes 8 hours to complete a hairstyle with extensions.

So it takes about eight hours to complete a box braid hairstyle that lasts for at least two months. See the third column "Extensions."

Once the style is complete, there is nominal maintenance time to take care of the braids. Washing the braids will only take 20 minutes since deep conditioning is not recommended for extensions styles. Daily and nightly preparations take only one minute. Taking the braids out is the most time-consuming part of wearing braids. But even so:

a person with extension braids barely spends 25 hours on hair care bimonthly.

You can do the math for the other two hairstyles however, the message should be clear. The schedule proves that although it is time-consuming to create natural hairstyles; the daily and weekly maintenance of chemically altered hair takes much more time than natural hair care. Even with exaggerating untangling times in the natural hair columns. In fact, relaxed hair maintenance always consumes more time than caring for natural hair.

Conclusion

Hopefully, by explaining the basic stubborn misconceptions, you will be able to separate facts from fiction. Being able to separate the two is an important part of journey. It means that you are ready and open to see the beautiful truth about natural Afrikan hair.

Afrikan hair

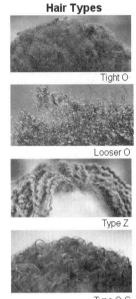

Characteristics

The most outstanding feature of Afrikan hair is its texture. The tightly coiled spiral ringlets separate Afrikan hair from other hair types at the first glance, and these coils vary in size as well as in form. The coils can have an O, S or Z form, and you can have a tight O, or S, or Z form, a loose O, S, or Z form, and anything in between. It is also very common to see more than one of these textures on the same head of hair.

The kinky, coiled and spiral ringlets that are so unique in Afrikan hair are also responsible for other unique characteristics. These characteristics may not be noticeable at one glance, but they do distinguish Afrikan hair from other hair types.
The characteristics are:

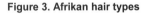

Figure 3. Afrikan hair types

~ its tenderness,

~ the tendency to group together,

~ the ability to absorb considerable moisture,

~ its matte look and,

~ the ability to shrink more than any other hair type.

Afrikan hair is tender

Afrikan hair is the most delicate of all hair types and the distinctive kinks and coils are responsible for the tenderness of this hair type. Everywhere a hair strand twists into a coil is, in fact, a vulnerable spot in the hair shaft. The tinier the coils, the sharper the angle in the hair strand and the more vulnerable the hair type. Too much stretching and bending may lead to a crack in the hair shaft right on the fragile spot, a crack that eventually will cause a hair strand to break. That is the reason why Afrikan hair is so vulnerable.

Afrikan hair densely groups together

Afrikan hair grows out of the scalp in different directions in spiral ringlets. Consequently, hair strands densely cover the scalp. This is a wonderful trait because we love having our scalp completely covered by hair. Conversely, however, there is some inconvenience connected to this trait. Hair that grows in different directions and densely packs together also tangles easily. The spiral curls are not symmetric so disturbed hair strands can hardly avoid each other on their way to their natural position and the coiled ringlets get tangled in each other.

Afrikan hair needs moisture

Afrikan hair thrives on moisture; kinks can only flourish when they are well-moisturized. To keep the kinks moisturized, Afrikan hair produces three times as much sebum as other hair types. Sebum is the grease that hair naturally produces to protect and lubricate the strands. However, the more the coils have to endure, the more moisture they need and the naturally produced sebum can quickly be insufficient because almost anything can disturb the moisture balance of the tender curls. Extreme weather conditions, synthetic products and heat can all draw moisture out of a coil, leaving the kinks feeling dry. Every time this happens, the moisture balance needs to be restored so that the coils can re-establish themselves. So, always keep your kinks moisturized; remember, water is your hair's best friend. Kinks can absorb loads of moisture and moisturized, natural hair is flexible; the kinks can stretch and bend without causing damage to the hair strands. For more about hair structure, see Appendix A.

Be careful of hard water

As much as our coils need water, be aware that hard water doesn't improve hair's health. We speak about hard water if it is high in minerals, normally calcium and magnesium. Hard water leaves a sticky residue that coats hair strands, leaving them feeling dry, hard and unmanageable. You know the film that develops over time in the sink or the bathtub? That same sticky residue can coat your hair and scalp and it may be the cause of your itchy scalp.

If you want to know whether you have hard water you can ask your water supplier about the hardness level or you can buy a water hardness testing kit at your local hardware store.

The easiest solution to the problems that come with hard water is a water treatment system for the shower. It will make a world of difference in the softness and manageability of your hair. You can buy a purification system at your local hardware store.

Dry versus matte

Another typical characteristic of Afrikan hair is that it is matte-looking. Natural Afrikan hair does not reflect light, which is why the hair has more of a matte sheen than a shiny look. People may confuse this with the hair being dry, which is something very different. Afrikan hair will not only feel dry if it is not well moisturized, it will also be fragile. Well-moisturized coils and kinks also absorb light, but the hair won't feel dry; it will be pliable rather than fragile.

Shrinkage

Shrinkage is very typical for Afrikan hair. Kinks are able to shrink anywhere from 20 to 80 percent. Shrinkage has everything to do with moisture. For instance, humid weather will cause the coils to shrink because the coils absorb the moisture of the humidity. The more moisture the coils are able to retain, the more the hair is able to shrink. With moisture and shrinkage comes frizz. Frizz is just inconsistent shrinkage of the kinks. To describe these two factors we can use the terms: cottony, wiry, spongy, wispy and thready.

Cottony – fine threads, 50 percent shrinkage or more, high frizz
Spongy – medium to thick threads, 65 percent shrinkage or more, high frizz
Wiry – thick threads, shrinkage varies, low frizz
Wispy – fine threads, shrinkage varies, low frizz
Thready – thick texture, low shrinkage, low frizz

Cottony hair is mostly fine textured with a shrinkage factor of about 50 percent or more. This hair type is high in frizz, quickly absorbs water but it takes time before hair is soaking wet.

Spongy hair with a medium to thick texture has a shrinkage factor of roughly 65 percent or more. This hair type has a compacted looking frizz and is able to absorb a lot of water before it gets thoroughly wet.

Wiry hair texture usually has thick threads and either high or low frizz. It seems as if hair never gets fully wet as if water bounces off the hair strands.

Wispy hair is fine-textured hair that easily blows in the wind because it is so light. It easily wets in water and either has a lot or low frizz.

Thready hair texture is usually thick with low frizz. Wets easily but water dries out quickly.

General hair characteristics and definitions

Like other hair types, Afrikan hair can be thick, thin, dense or not dense. The following definitions are generally used. They describe characteristics of all hair types and are not exclusive to Afrikan hair.

Thickness

The thickness of hair literally means the thickness of a hair strand. This is determined by the diameter of a hair strand. Hair strands can be fine, medium or course. Compare your hair to the thickness of a regular thread to find out how thick your strands are. Your hair strands are fine or thin if they are smaller in diameter size than a thread that is split in half, medium if they are the same size and thick if they are larger in diameter.

Density

The density of hair is literally the number of hair strands that a person has on his or her head. Although Afrikan hair always looks dense, density varies because not everyone with kinky hair has the same quantity of strands. Normally a person has 100,000 to 150,000 hair strands. This number of hair strands is determined for each of us individually by the time we are born. There seems to be a correlation between thickness and density: the thinner the hair strands, the denser the hair and the thicker the hair strands, the fewer number of hairs on the scalp. It could be hard to notice the difference in density because kinky hair strands naturally pack densely together, whether hair is fine, medium or thick.

Hair growth

In general, people assume that Afrikan hair can't grow long. However, there is no scientific evidence that supports this statement. In fact, dreadlocks are proof that Afrikan hair can grow long. Hair type does not determine hair growth, genes do. Genes determine hair growth and length and they do so for each individual. Diet does influence hair growth. The foods we eat affect our hair growth the same way good or poor nutrition affect a child's growth. Every child has the potential to grow and reach a certain height, but good nutrition is essential for the child to reach his or her maximum size in a healthy way. Hormones also influence hair growth. Most pregnant women will notice thicker and longer hair growth. For more about biological hair growth, see Appendix A.

Afrikan hair	Straight hair
Has curls, kinks and coils	Is just straight
Absorbs light	Reflects light
Grows up	Grows down
Stands up	Lays down
Shrinks	Hardly shrinks
Excellent for braiding styles	Poor for braiding styles

Table 2 Afrikan hair vs. straight hair

Hair breakage

Hair breakage is one of the biggest issues in Afrikan hair care. It is the main reason why Afrikan hair does not grow long; the tender hair strands break before they get a chance to reach their maximum length. To be able to reach our maximum hair length, we have to prevent our hair from breaking. To keep our hair from breaking, we have to look at the causes of hair breakage.

Hair breaking factors

Afrikan hair is tender, but that does not mean that our hair is doomed to break. For the most part, we are responsible for the breakage of our hair. We have some damaging habits that destroy our kinks. If we want our hair to stop breaking and gain length, we need to stop these damaging habits and work on routines that cherish our natural naps.

CHEMICALS
Chemicals are bad regardless the hair type. Relaxers, coloring and perms are all damaging to hair. On top of this, women of color with naturally tender hair are using these harmful chemicals too easily and too often. This leads to split ends, hair breakage and hair loss. If you're suffering from hair breakage, and you want to grow healthy hair, stop using any of these chemicals. To know more about the way relaxers work, see Appendix B.

HEAT

The heat appliances we use so freely to style our hair can cause severe damage to our naps. Curling irons, press combs and blow dryers are all capable of producing enough heat to harm our kinks. By using these tools repeatedly, hair becomes lifeless, dull and is likely to develop split ends. The heat disturbs the moisture balance and damages the outer layer of a hair shaft. This results in a reshaped pattern of the natural ringlets and once they are damaged, the hair may never return to its original texture.

INAPPROPRIATE BRAIDING

Despite what people believe, braiding is not the cause of hair breakage - *inappropriate* braiding is: Braids are, in so many ways, excellent for Afrikan hair. Not only do they adorn the hair, braids can also stimulate hair growth if the job is done well. Inappropriate braiding on the other hand has terrible consequences. Braids that are too tight or micro-braids are disastrous for one's hair. You can read more on braiding in Chapter 3.

INAPPROPRIATE HAIR CARE

In spite of all the love for our hair, many of us inappropriately care for it. Not only are our hair care methods wrong, we also often use the wrong tools and the wrong products. By using the wrong tools, we damage the kinks and that leads to breakage. Using the wrong types of products only adds to damage instead of fixing it. The next chapter discusses appropriate Afrikan hair care.

Afrikan hair care

Appropriate hair care is essential to give any hair type a chance to flourish. The best hair care is care that is tailored to the hair type. Since Afrikan hair is known to be tender, the standard for good Afrikan hair care is:

Tender hair needs gentle products, gentle tools and tender care.

Hair products

The market for Afrikan hair products is booming; there are numerous products available. The supply is only growing and the availability for natural hair is clearly increasing. That is a good thing but it doesn't make finding the right products easier. In this health conscious era, we as customers are much more aware of the products we buy and consume and going natural will only fortify this. This means that you won't just look for a product that might work for you. You'll want to make sure that the product won't harm your natural kinks but will nurture them. Thus, you'll be interested in the ingredients are used in any hair product you purchase.

Product labels
The world of cosmetic ingredients is a fairly complicated one. Only a fraction of the synthetic components have thoroughly been tested but most of them are still presumed safe until proven harmful[1]. The problem with this is that it's hard to say how safe or dangerous synthetic ingredients are. Some may be a threat to our health but some may not and it's not unlikely to have two contradicting stories about the same ingredient. Like the Rio relaxer[2] it usually takes dramatic injuries and public outcry to ban a product or ingredient. Unfortunately, at that point, the harm has been done. Currently, the best thing one can do is educate oneself on the subject of cosmetic ingredients and learn to read the labels. This can help you select better products for your hair as well as for your entire body. Hopefully it will also prevent disasters like the one mentioned above.

Ingredients
Ingredients are normally listed in the order of their concentrations within the product. Few products have their ingredients listed alphabetically. If they are, it should be mentioned on the package. In general, the one percent rule applies. This means that one can assume that ingredients listed on the top half of a label are included in concentrations above one percent or more and the ones below in less than one percent.

For example, in the listing below, water is first ingredient and fragrance the last. This would mean that it's a water-based product that contains less than one percent fragrance.

Ingredients:

Water, Cetyl Alcohol, Stearyl Alcohol, Cyclomethicone, Stearyl Octyldimonium Methosulfate, Panthenol, Hair Keratin Amino Acids, Hydroxyethylcellulose, Citric Acid, Stearamidopropyl Dimethylamine, Behenamidopropyl Ethyldimonium Ethosulfate, Disodium EDTA, Methylchloroisothiazolinone, Methylisothiazolinone, DMDM Hydantoin, Amodimethicone, Tallowtrimonium Chloride, Nonoxynol-10, Fragrance

---

Ingredients to avoid

A search on the Internet using the keywords "unsafe cosmetic ingredients" will provide you with several lists of beauty agents that you should avoid[3] but at the same time you will find websites that contradict or mitigate the use of the listed agents. None of the ingredients are prohibited by the Food and Drug Administration (FDA) or the Cosmetic, Toiletry and Fragrance Association (CFTA[4]) but there are recommended limitations for their uses. Maybe that proves that the ingredients are unsafe or maybe not. Since there is still controversy about them it might be better to avoid the following ingredients until they are thoroughly tested and proven completely safe.

1. *Sodium Lauryl Sulfate (SLS) And Sodium Laureth Sulfate (SLES)*
Sodium Lauryl Sulfate is a popular ingredient used in many personal-care products. In hair formulas it's mainly used in shampoos as a detergent and a surfactant. It strongly decreases and dries out the hair strands and causes eye irritations[5]. The CFTA has an alert for this ingredient on their website and recommends that concentrations should not exceed one percent.
Sodium Laureth Sulfate (SLES) is milder than SLS, but may be more drying than SLS and it also contains ether[6].

2. *Propylene Glycol*
This ingredient is used as a humectant[ξ], surfactant or solvent in several cosmetics like shampoos and hair conditioners and also in skin and beauty creams. It can cause allergic and toxic reactions if used in concentrations of more than five percent[7].

[ξ] See Glossary

3. *Mineral oil and Petrolatum*
Mineral oil is used in a wide variety of hair and skin products as an emollient. It is a petrochemical by-product that coats the skin and keeps it from breathing naturally. As a consequence, it dries out the skin rather than moisturize it. It is known to be comedogenic[ξ]. Petrolatum is mineral oil jelly and has the same effects. [8]

4. *TEA (triethanolamine)*
TEA is used in various cosmetics as a pH balancer. It can cause allergic reactions and dryness to hair and skin if used in concentrations of more than five percent. Absorption may be toxic with prolonged use. [9]

5. *Imidazolidinyl Urea and Diazolidinyl Urea*
Imidazolidinyl Urea is commonly used as a preservative in shampoos and is known to cause contact dermatitis (American Academy of Dermatology).
Diazolidinyl Urea is a disinfectant that is used as a moisturizer in hair preparations and other cosmetics and may cause contact dermatitis. [10]

6. *Synthetic Fragrances*
Fragrances are virtually present in all cosmetic products from shampoos to baby products and conceal the smell of the ingredients. Nearly all synthetic fragrances contain toxic ingredients that can cause sneezing, headaches, dizziness, rashes, skin discoloration, coughing and vomiting, and allergic skin irritation. Natural scents from plants or essential oils are generally safer. [11]

7. *Synthetic Color additives and hair dye*
There is a great deal of controversy about the use of synthetic colors. Not only in hair dyes and other hair products, but also in food, drugs and cosmetics. According to *A Consumer's Dictionary of Cosmetic Ingredients* many pigments can cause skin sensitivity and irritation and studies have shown nearly all of the colors made from coal tar are carcinogenic in animals. Since it's unclear which ones are unsafe, it might be best to avoid synthetic colors altogether. [12]

8. *Parabens: Methylparaben, Propylparaben and Butylparaben*
Parabens have anti-microbial properties and are used as preservatives to

---

[ξ] Clog pores

extend shelf life of moisturizers, shampoos and cleansers. They are widely used, but they can cause allergic reactions and skin rashes if the concentration exceeds the level of five percent[13].

9. *Alcohol*
Ethanol, denatured alcohol, ethyl alcohol, methanol, benzyl alcohol, isopropyl, and SD alcohol are the types of alcohols you want to avoid. They are used in a range of cosmetic products such as solvents or carrying agents, but they can be drying and irritating to scalp[14].

10. *Formaldehyde*
Formaldehyde is used as a disinfectant or preservative in a wide variety of cosmetics including hair products. It is a colorless, pungent substance that is suspected to be carcinogenic[15].

Ingredients to look for
Not all ingredients are bad. Fortunately, there are also ingredients that can help us nurture our hair. Next is a list of ingredients that can help protect, moisturize and condition our kinks. Be aware that even though an ingredient is known to be beneficial in hair care, it may not benefit you at all if you are allergic to it. If you are sensitive to any one of these agents, avoid them in your hair care as well.

1. *Aloe vera*
Aloe, native to Africa, also referred to as "lily of the desert," the "plant of immortality," and the "medicine plant," is one of the oldest medicinal plants known. The name was derived from the Arabic word "alloeh," meaning "bitter," because of the taste of the liquid in the leaves and already in 1500 B.C. Egyptians recorded use of the herbal plant in treating burns, infections and parasites.
Aloe vera is a rich emollient that promotes the healing of damaged or dry hair and skin. It is a natural oxygenator[ξ] that acts as a moisturizer, soother and nutrient in various hair and other cosmetic formulas.

2. *Shea butter*
Shea butter is also referred to as "women's gold" in Afrikan communities because of its healing and cosmetic qualities that have been valued for centuries. References as early as Cleopatra's Egypt mention caravans bearing clay jars of Shea butter cosmetic use.

[ξ] drawing and holding oxygen to the skin

This vegetable butter made from Shea nuts from the Karite tree that grows in West Afrika has restructuring effects on dry and fragile hair. It is an excellent emollient that softens the coils, makes them more pliable and protects the hair strands.

3. *Jojoba oil*
Jojoba oil is actually a liquid wax derived from the seeds of the small woody Jojoba tree. Native Americans have used pure jojoba oil for centuries for its cosmetic and medical qualities. This odorless liquid is virtually identical to sebum, the oil our scalp naturally produces, and can easily be absorbed by hair and scalp. Jojoba lubricates the hair shafts. If there is too much sebum buildup on the scalp, it dissolves the sebum, leaving the hair clean. It is a highly effective cleanser, conditioner, moisturizer, and softener for hair and skin.

4. *MSM*
MSM is an organic type of sulfur that naturally occurs in ocean organisms called phytoplankton, but it's also in fresh foods and vegetables as well as in the human body. Supplements of MSM are used for a variety of aliments from allergies to arthritis and also to improve overall heath. In hair care, MSM is used in anti-dandruff formulas because of its anti-inflammatory qualities. Since it is known to improve the condition of hair and skin, you will find it in conditioners to soften and strengthen hair.

5. *Natural herbs*
Plants or parts of them have always been valued for their medicinal, savory, or aromatic qualities and they reclaimed their popularity in today's society where "organic" and "natural" are keywords in marketing. Rosemary, sage, lavender, nettle and horsetail extract are just some of the common herbs you are likely to see labeled on hair products. They are all beneficial in their own ways. Rosemary and nettle are known to nourish and stimulate hair growth, sage and lavender have natural cleansing and reviving properties and horsetail helps normalize and balance the skin and scalp.

6. *Vegetable proteins*
Proteins are called "the building blocks of life," because every cell in our bodies depends on proteins, thus, the reason they are so essential in our diet. It is used in various cosmetics, however, because external use of this complex structure can also benefit hair and skin. Hair is made out of a certain protein called keratin, and proteins obtained from plant sources like

wheat germ and soy coat porous or damaged hair and split-ends. Soy protein adds a protective layer to the hair shaft that seals in moisture.

7. *Vegetable glycerine*
Vegetable glycerine is a clear, colorless, and odorless liquid with a very sweet taste that is naturally extracted from vegetable oils. This thick syrup-like liquid is used in various cosmetics as a humectant, emollient and lubricant. It is often used in conditioners and styling agents to soften and soothe (should this be smooth?) the hair strands and help them to retain moisture.

8. *Panthenol*
Panthenol, known for its revitalizing and conditioning effects, is used in shampoos and conditioners to add moisture and volume to hair strands. This agent binds well to hair follicles and attracts moisture from the air, which helps to give hair body and hold. Panthenol also smoothes roughened hair surfaces, making them shiny and easier to comb. It hydrates the scalp as well.

9. *Biotin*
Biotin is a type of vitamin B-complex also known as vitamin H. It is used in hair formulas to add body and shine and also to promote hair growth and prevent hair loss.

10.   *Cholesterol*
Although it is known as the type of fat you want to avoid in your diet, our natural hair oil sebum, is high in cholesterol and it may be beneficial in hair products. It can be obtained from animals as well as from plants like cocoa beans and is used as emulsifier and lubricant in a variety of cosmetic formulas.

A few more hints
Some of us may want to buy products that are natural, hypoallergenic or even safety tested for obvious personal reasons. Your idea of what these words mean may be different from reality. According to the FDA's website, http://www.fda.gov/, there are no official government definitions for the terms like fragrance-free, hypoallergenic and natural.

Fragrance-free or unscented
Products with these labels may still contain small amounts of fragrances to mask or neutralize the unpleasant odors of the basic ingredients they contains.

Hypoallergenic
The definition of this term is: "Cosmetics that are less likely to cause allergic reactions."
"Less likely" doesn't exclude allergic reactions.

Natural and organic
Some products claim to be "natural" or "organic" but only contain one natural or organic component so these terms really don't say anything about the quality of cosmetics.

Cruelty free or not tested on animals
Maybe the product itself has not been tested on animals but it is very likely that the ingredients have. It will take more years before the process of shifting testing from animals to alternative methods is in place.

Dermatology tested
A test from one dermatologist on one person makes this a truthful statement but this doesn't mean that the product is safe.

The right products
The previous lists are, by far, neither absolute nor complete. They are guidelines to help you find your way through the overwhelming supply in product land. Learning to read the labels puts you halfway to finding the right products. This is, in fact, a very personal choice because everybody has different needs and different tastes. Some people like light concoctions while others prefer heavy or medium products, so it is impossible to have one formula that will work for everyone. Product recommendations are great but don't feel disappointed if a product that seems to work for everybody else doesn't work for you. The right product is one that works for you and, in the end, you decide which one suits you best.

PJ's rehabilitate
PJ stands for product junkie and it is used for those of us who are addicted to buying and trying a thousand products at the same time. Although it could be a lot of fun experimenting with so many different formulas and brands, it is not necessary. Besides the golden rule, "Tender hair needs gentle products," there is another saying that applies to tender hair care: "Less is more." You don't need to use a dozen products to care for your naps; this won't improve their health. Using too many products at the same time causes buildup, which will only add extra time to your hair care routine because you have to get rid of more residue more frequently or it might stiffen and damage your

strands. So in fact, too many products will only cost you extra time and money. The truth is, you don't have to spend much money to keep your hair healthy. Ordinary, natural products that are common in one's household, like olive oil, often work as good as commercial products. This is especially great for people on a budget. You can read more on this subject in the paragraph "natural hair care." First, let's take a look at common products in today's hair care.

Shampoos

The use of shampoos is overrated. Shampoos are a product of the industrial revolution times when people who worked in factories needed something to break down the heavy dirt and grease after a hard day's labor. By the end of industrial revolution, shampoos were marketed as the way to keep the hair clean in an affluent society that was obsessed with hygiene. Commercials full of marvelous bubbles let us believe that shampoo was indispensable for civilized families for aesthetic reasons. Like most commercials, those that promoted shampoos were also designed to sell illusions rather than stating facts. The sebum and perspiration that the scalp produces are sterile, clean and necessary to protect the scalp. Our hair needs cleaning from pollution, residue and bacteria and even though shampoos are a lot milder today, they are still designed to emulsify fats and oils and most of them are still too harsh for our natural naps. They strip the naps from their natural oils leaving the hair feeling dry. For this reason, it may be better to do the no-poo or condition-wash method[16] discussed in the next paragraph.

If you wish to use shampoo, look for an herbal shampoo, a shampoo that is pH-balanced or one that does not contain these harsh ingredients: Sodium Lauryl Sulfate, Ammonium Laureth Sulfate or Sodium Laureth Sulfate. The last ingredient is a little gentler but avoiding it is recommended.

No-poo or conditioning-wash

As an alternative to the use of shampoos, Lorraine Massey introduced the conditioning-wash method in her book "Curly Girl". It means washing hair with a conditioner to avoid the harsh ingredients of common shampoos. Most conditioners also contain cleaning agents and washing your hair with them cleans the strands without stripping them of their moisture. After it was posted on the forum of Nappturality[ξ], many visitors adopted the method and named it "No-poo."

[ξ] http://nappturality.com

Conditioners

Conditioners are essential in Afrikan hair for several reasons:
They clean the naps without stripping them of their moisture,
They improve the manageability of strands, and
They replenish moisture and lubricate the hair strands from the inside out.

Not all conditioners are the same; there are different types which serve different purposes. There are three categories: instant, leave-in, deep and reconstructing conditioners.

Instant conditioners

Instant conditioners are all conditioners that need to be rinsed out instantly within one to three minutes. Daily reconstructive, moisturizing, hydrating conditioners, and other similar formulas are all instant conditioners and their collective purpose is to soften and smooth the hair strands, which makes them excellent detanglers.

These conditioners are ideal for no-pooing: to use as a shampoo to wash the hair. Unlike most shampoos, instant conditioners clean the hair without stripping the coils from their natural moisture. Not all conditioners should be used to clean hair. Instant and leave-in conditioners are usually good to no-poo but deep conditioners and reconstructing conditioners should be used for their stated purposes.

Leave-in conditioners

Leave-in conditioners are also good detangling agents but the difference is that they don't need to be rinsed out and they can be used as a daily moisturizer. A disadvantage is that they coat the hair shaft and can cause buildup over time, so be careful.

Deep conditioners

Deep conditioners are designed to improve the condition of one's hair by replenishing moisture, lubricating and strengthening the strands. Unlike the crème and instant conditioners, deep conditioners don't just stay on the surface of a hair shaft, they penetrate the hair shaft. That's why they should remain in the hair for at least 20 minutes. Usually heat is recommended to promote penetration. Always follow the directions for use and rinse hair thoroughly after deep conditioning. Residue can harden the hair shaft, making the strands inflexible and prone to breakage.

Reconstructing conditioners

Reconstructing conditioners are designed to repair and strengthen damaged hair. To be effective they should remain in the hair for at least 20 minutes. Be very careful with these types of conditioners. They contain concentrated levels of protein that can harm hair that is already extremely dry and brittle if they are not rinsed out well. Therefore, it is better to leave protein treatments to professionals. If your hair breakage is caused by extreme dryness of your strands, a deep conditioner that is designed to moisturize your hair is probably better.

Detanglers
Detanglers are slippery emulsions primarily designed to untangle hair without damaging the strands. They contain emollients that increase the manageability which eases knots and snarls and leave the strands feeling silky.
Detanglers are often instant conditioners, but they also come as leave-in conditioners or other styling products that can either be used on wet or dry hair.

Moisturizers
Moisturizers are excellent humectants$^{\xi}$. They keep the curls supple by adding moisture and some oily substances to the hair shafts. Moisturizers are preferable over grease because they penetrate the hair shafts, while most types of grease just coat the hair making the naps look greasy rather than allowing them to shine. A good moisturizer doesn't make the hair look or feel greasy, nor does it weigh down the naps.
There are countless moisturizers available at any beauty supply store. Try to find a light one that your hair absorbs and avoid the ones that coat and dry out the hair.

Pomades
Pomades are especially designed for kinky and curly hair to provide hold, shine and control. They are mainly used on short and medium-length hair to give form and definition and to smooth hair. Many types of pomade are greasy and contain wax so they are difficult to wash out of your hair.

Hair butters
Hair butters are conditioners designed to provide hold, shine and control. Unlike pomades, they don't stiffen the hair but they leave hair soft and not greasy as pomades do. Hair butters are usually solid, rich substances based

---

$^{\xi}$ See Glossary

on natural butters like cocoa and Shea butter and most of them can be used as a pre- or post-wash conditioning treatment.

Styling gels

Gels add shine and fight frizz, but they provide little hold to Afrikan hair. They soften and add moisture to the kinks and are often used to control frizz and to smooth the hair. Silicone-based gels are supposed to fight frizz by blocking humidity. Before you buy a gel, try it on your skin first; if it feels sticky, it will make your hair sticky. Some gels even make your hair feel crunchy after they dry. Also, choose a colorless gel without alcohol. Colored gels leave a film over the strands and alcohol has a drying effect on our naps.

Natural hair care

Natural hair products are usually more expensive than typical commercial ones, and they are often harder to find but they can be worth the effort. Most of them are free from fragrances and other synthetic ingredients, which reduces the possibility of allergic reactions like itchy scalp. Carefully read the labels before you spend extra money on a product that is labeled as natural. If you want to use natural products but you don't want to spend extra money there is a simpler solution. Common natural stuff that's usually available in most kitchens can be as nurturing to our naps as commercial hair products. Actually, using daily foodstuff as hair aids has two advantages - it is cheaper and 100 percent natural.

Shea butter

Shea butter, the natural butter mentioned in the list of "Ingredients to look for," is excellent for most Afrikan hair types in its purest form. One hundred percent Shea butter softens the coils, makes them more pliable and protects the hair strands. It is a rich, solid substance that softens when you rub it in your hands and melts on a hot summer day. You can either use it on wet or dry hair and a little goes a long way.

Pure Shea butter can most easily be purchased in Afrikan stores or online because not many beauty supplies have it in their inventory. Be aware that there are products that claim to be 100 percent Shea butter, but in fact, they are refined, which means that the Shea butter is bleached and probably has fragrance added to it. Some people prefer the refined formula because they prefer the scent over that of the natural Shea butter.

Oils

Natural oils are wonderful for Afrikan hair. They are good emollients; they lubricate and protect our strands. Using natural oils as hot oil treatments are often as good as commercial deep conditioners. These treatments are excellent to moisturize and lubricate our naps.

Coconut oil

Coconut oil is one of the best oils one can use on natural hair. It softens, detangles and it is a wonderful hair conditioner. Beauticians who are familiar with this oil swear by it. Coconut oil is also used as a pre-wash conditioner to help against dandruff. Another benefit of this oil is its quality to strengthen the structure of damaged, devitalized hair.

The best way to purchase coconut oil is at a supermarket. They probably have the same quality as the health store, but the price is more competitive. Make sure to choose the pure coconut oil, that is, the one you can use for cooking without any additional chemical ingredients.

Jojoba oil

Native Americans have used pure jojoba oil for centuries for its cosmetic and medicinal properties. Pure jojoba oil is virtually identical to sebum, the oil our scalp naturally produces. It is a light oil that can easily be absorbed by hair and scalp. Jojoba lubricates the hair shafts, and if there is too much sebum buildup on the scalp, it dissolves the sebum, leaving the hair clean. This quality makes jojoba oil ideal for extension hairstyles. It is a highly effective cleanser, conditioner, moisturizer, and softener for hair and skin.

Olive oil

Olive oil is easy to use because it is widely available and relatively cheap compared to hair products we buy. Olive oil smooths and softens (an emollient) with penetrating ability. It also has the ability to nourish, condition, and improve the strength and elasticity of hair. After a long winter's exposure to dry, indoor heat, a hot Olive oil treatment can give your hair some nourishing relief.

Like the coconut oil, the best way to purchase Olive oil is at a supermarket where it's also cheaper than buying in a health food store. Make sure it's pure olive oil but it doesn't have to be extra virgin if you don't use it to cook. Some people don't like the strong scent, and as long as it is for cosmetic purposes, you don't need the most expensive one.

Cold press means that the process to make the oil is done without heat or chemicals.

Fully ripe is produced by crushing the pulp of the fruit and not the seed, and different qualities are available and range from extra virgin, virgin and pure. Pomace is the ground flesh and pits after pressing. Any oil that hasn't been removed by pressure can then be extracted using steam and solvents. This kind is used for soap-making or industrial purposes.

Tea tree oil

Australian aboriginals have used tea tree leaves for centuries to help heal skin conditions as well as for other health purposes. This oil is anti-fungal, anti-septic and anti-bacterial, which is why it is used to combat dandruff and other scalp maladies. Tea tree oil is also recommended to keep the scalp clean free from bacteria. Many hair products today contain tea tree oil to smooth and to control an itchy scalp.

Castor   oil

This is a very thick oil with a pungent odor and a slightly sticky texture. It is used mainly for hair conditions such as dry, brittle, damaged hair or hair loss and as a hair conditioner.

The oil, when used in cosmetics, acts as a humectant; it attracts and retains moisture to the skin. It is also a thickener and an emollient.

Other oils

Most vegetables and nut oils like avocado, almond and castor oil can be used to nourish natural hair or as a hot oil treatment. Some people use them in conjunction with other products. For example, they may add a little oil to a conditioner. Be careful oiling your scalp because most oils are comedogenic, which means they can clog your pores.

Natural nurturing

Using homemade recipes to nurture one's hair is as old as humankind. When the overwhelming supply of the hair care industry offered easier alternatives, the recipes went out of favor but now they regained popularity. With an increasing health awareness, more consumers favor natural ingredients and even the hygiene companies are looking at the "old" homemade formulas. These out-of-style but never forgotten recipes have proven to be excellent treatments for hair. They are easy to make because the necessary ingredients are usually in one's kitchen.

Coconut Oil Pre Conditioning Treatment

¼ cup of honey
¼ cup of coconut oil

Pastry brush (optional)
Shower or conditioning cap[ξ]

Mix the honey and the coconut oil in a cup placed in hot water. Use the pastry brush to work the warm mixture through the hair section by section until the hair is fully coated. Cover hair with a shower cap; leave on 30 minutes. No-poo and rinse well.

This treatment is ideal for damaged and dry hair with split ends. Honey is a natural humectant that draws moisture into the hair shafts and seals it in. You can also mix equal parts of honey with your favorite deep conditioner. It is also possible to substitute coconut oil with olive oil or another one of your favorite oils. Essential oils can also be added to the hot oil treatment to enhance the effects.

Just mayo
½ cup of mayonnaise
3 drops essential oil of your choice
Conditioning or shower cap

Mayonnaise is an excellent conditioner for dry hair. Add a few drops of your favorite essential oil to approximately half a cup depending on the length of your hair. Saturate your hair with mayonnaise before it is wet. When it is worked well into the hair, cover hair with the conditioning cap and allow the mayonnaise to set for about 15 minutes. Rinse thoroughly and then wash hair as usual.

Banana/Avocado conditioner
½ a ripe banana
½ a cup of ripe avocado
1 tablespoon olive oil
1 egg yolk

Mix all the ingredients in a blender until they are very well blended. The mixture should almost be like a liquid puree. Massage the mixture into your hair, and especially your scalp, after washing your hair. Cover hair with a conditioning cap for 45 minutes to an hour. Don't use heat and rinse with room temperature to warm water or your hair will be adorned with

---

[ξ] This is not a heating cap. It's like a shower cap from isolating material instead of plastic

scrambled egg. Follow with a baking soda or apple cider vinegar (ACV) rinse; you can find the recipes for these rinses in the next paragraph. This beauty recipe is worth keeping, as it revitalizes the hair and makes it shiny and healthy looking.

Easy does it conditioning treatment
¼ cup aloe vera gel
½ of a lemon
3-5 drops essential oils of your choice

This is an easy natural conditioner ideal for of dry, damaged and brittle hair. Mix the gel with the juice and add a couple of drops of your favorite essential oil. Apply the mixture to freshly washed hair, leave it on for three to five minutes and then rinse thoroughly.

Natural Rinses
Using natural rinses after no-pooing is a treat for the hair. These rinses eliminate the previous product's remains. They also add shine and nutrition to one's hair while leaving the hair soft.

Clarifying baking soda rinse
1 tablespoon of baking soda
1 cup warm spring water
Spray bottle

Add the baking soda and the water to the spray bottle and shake until the baking soda is dissolved. Spray freely over the hair after no-pooing and let it set for one to three minutes before you rinse. This clarifying rinse is ideal for those who are using heavy grease products. It will effectively clean the hair of heavy product buildup while leaving the strands with a soft feeling.

Apple cider vinegar rinse (ACV)
1 cup of cool spring water
2 cups of apple cider vinegar
(preferably unfiltered non-pasteurized from the health food store)
Spray bottle

Mix the vinegar and the water in the spray bottle and freely spray after no-pooing. ACV restores moisture, removes residue and seals the hair shaft. It is very popular among people who wear dreadlocks.
Feel free to try pleasant-scented vinegar such as raspberry or plum or add jojoba oil and essential oils to leave a more moisturized feeling.

Natural spritzes
Spritzes mist the hair and are ideal to keep coils moisturized throughout the day. Kinks love moisture whether it is a hot summer day or a cold winter afternoon. Adding a couple drops of your favorite essential oil to boiled spring water easily makes a natural spritz that will keep your curls moist and your hair fresh all day. Try some of these essential oils:
Lavender - stimulates scalp, antibiotic, antiseptic and acts as a calming agent.
Rosemary - mild astringent that stimulates hair growth (Avoid during pregnancy)
Tea tree - soothing and cleansing agent that stimulates and irrigates scalp

Moisturizing spritz
1 teaspoon of aloe vera juice
1 teaspoon of vegetable glycerin (available at health food stores)
3 drops of your favorite essential oils
Spring water
Spray bottle

Bring the water to a boil and let it simmer for an hour to get rid of impurities. Add the ingredients, stir and let it steep until the mixture cools. Pour into the spray bottle and use it as a daily moisturizer to style and keep your hairstyle refreshed.

Styling spray
This styling spray was posted on Nappturality's website. It is ideal to keep crinkles in the hair, for instance, if one wants to wear a twist-out or a braid-out. It also keeps crinkles and curls in locs.

1.5 cup of spring water
2 tablespoons of olive oil
4 tablespoons of honey

Bring the water to a boil and let it simmer to release impurities. Add the ingredients, stir and let the mixture cool. Pour into spray bottle.

Nappturality's most popular hair growth spritz
A most popular natural solution on Nappturality to stimulate hair growth was the homemade Rosemary spray. Daily spraying on the scalp's problem areas seems to stimulate hair growth and fill in thinning spots. Many women were

very enthusiastic about this concoction but use wisely; Rosemary should not be used on women who are pregnant.

3-4 Rosemary tea bags
2-3 drops of sage essential oil
1-2 cups of water
Spray bottle

Bring the water to a boil and let it simmer to release impurities. Add the rosemary teabags and let it steep for about an hour. The more the bags steep, the more concentrated the brew will be. If it gets too concentrated the spritz may cause your scalp to itch. Add 2-3 drops of sage oil and pour in a spray bottle.

Keep the concoction sealed and refrigerated all the time to prevent it from going bad. Also use it within three weeks.

Gentle Hair Tools

Hands and fingers are by far the best tools one can use for grooming natural hair. It will take some time before you become skilled at it, but the more you learn to know your naps and the longer they grow, the more you will get used to using hands and fingers to groom your hair. One can smooth, style, braid, twist, untangle, untwist and unbraid the hair with only the hands. Until you reach that point, you will need a couple of other tools to help you to groom your kinks. Remember: use gentle tools on tender hair.

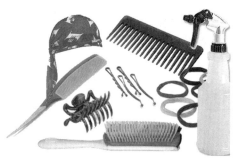

Figure 4. Hair tools

1. Tools to untangle
   Since untangling is a natural part of Afrikan hair care, selecting gentle tools to untangle it are crucial. Combs or brushes with sharp edges will

tear your naps. Wide tooth combs like the one in figure 4 can be found everywhere. Select one with rounded edges and anti-static material. Finding a good brush that untangles nappy hair without damaging it is a little harder. The most frequently recommended brushes among naturals and natural hair stylists are the Denman D3, D4 or D41 and the Goody classic rubber base brush which is similar to the Denman D41 type. These are half-round brushes with rounded nylon pins set into an anti-static natural rubber pad.

2. Night protection
Eight hours of sleep every night on a cotton pillowcase may dry out your hair. Satin and silk do not dry out your hair because they don't absorb the moisture that your hair needs to stay healthy. A silk do-rak is as good as a pillowcase. Another alternative is to tie a silk scarf on your pillow if you have problems keeping the scarf on your head while sleeping.

3. Styling
A rattail comb, pins, bobby pins and clips
If you want to do your own hairstyles, clips may be handy to keep the hair in place or parted while you style your hair. A rattail comb is handy to do the parting for most hairstyles like designer braids and coils. You will only need the tail, never the comb. Small toothed combs are not for natural hair.

4. Moisture
Since natural hair loves moisture, a spray bottle comes in very handy. Not only after washing to keep the hair wet while untangling and styling, but also to keep the hair moisturized and fresh after styling.

5. Adornments
Scarves, headbands, hats and other items are handy to adorn the hair and to provide protection from extreme temperatures, for instance, on a hot summer day while on the beach. Ponytail holders are very handy for bantus or afro-puffs. Use the brands that are made out of gentle material without metal parts. Metal parts can pull out, tangle or damage your naps and as can rubber bands.

Going-Natural Starter's Kit
Even with the provided information, it will be hard to find the right products and tools to start your natural journey. That's why *Going-Natural* offers a starter's kit. The kit is meant to help you to make a good start and consists of carefully selected nappy-friendly products that are approved by veteran naturals. It contains pure Afrikan Shea butter to soften your new growth, a

nappy-friendly hair brush to help you untangle and a concoction to strengthen the hair strands and prevent breakage during transitioning. You can order the starter's kit online at http://going-natural.com.

Tender hair care

Gentle products and gentle tools put us halfway towards the goal of appropriate Afrikan hair care. All we need is tender hair care to complete the regimen. Here are the basic guidelines for tender hair care to make your naps flourish.

Moisturize regularly

Since our tender curls thrive on moisture, using a moisturizer on a regular basis is essential to our hair care. This way the coils keep their pliability, and pliable hair does not easily break. In fact, keeping hair moisturized will keep the coils from breaking so that hair can bloom and reach its maximum length.

Minimize tangles

The best way to handle tangles is to minimize them. Minimizing tangles will not only reduce the amount of tangles but will also make it easier to take the tangles out. These simple rules will help minimize tangles if your hair is longer than three inches.

~ Completely untangle hair before creating a new lasting hairstyle like cornrows, coils, braids.

~ Keep hair in braids or twists as much as possible.

~ Untangle hair after washing before it dried.

~ If you wear your hair out, braid or twist hair before going to bed.

~ Do not go sleep on tangled or wet hair.

~ Keep hair moist; dry curls tangle easier

The art of untangling

Since it is inevitable for lively coils to intertwine, we need to know how to correctly untangle our hair strands. We should master the art of untangling to be able to untie knots without damaging or breaking hair strands. It will take some practice, and a little patience, but once you know how to do it, you'll wonder what the fuss was all about.

Time and patience

Always take the time to untangle your hair. Don't start doing it if you are in a hurry. Your kinks will only suffer from impatient and hasty pulling; the knots will get tighter and there is a likely chance that you'll do damage to your hair. All this will only upset you and won't contribute to your happiness or beauty. That's reason enough to take your time.

Sectioning

Don't try to comb your entire head at once unless you have some freshly cut naps of one inch or less. Forget about the commercials where you see women combing through their long, thick hair with one stroke; it just doesn't work like that. Not for anyone. Always work in sections. If your hair is between two and four inches long, you can section and untangle at the same time. If your hair has passed four inches, it's easier to create sections before you start to untangle.

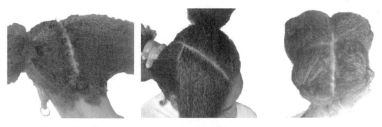

Figure 5. Parting the hair

Here is an easy way to part your hair into sections. You need a rattail comb and either clips or scrunchies. If your hair is long enough you won't need clips or scrunchies, you can twirl or twist each section and tuck it in its base to keep separated hair place. Remember, don't comb or brush while sectioning, just use your fingers to separate the parts and strands from each other.

1. Put the tail of the comb in the middle of your front hairline and carefully start parting. The tail won't go through at once. If it gets caught up in a couple of kinks, stop and separate the hair with your fingers before continuing to part. Carry on until your hair is divided in a left and a right part.

2. Gather one part and secure it with a scrunchie or separate it with clips from the other part.
3. Take the other loose part and divide it into 2 parts. Start with the rattail in the middle of your head and carefully pull in a straight line to the top of your ear. Again stop if the tail doesn't go through at once and separate the hair with your hands.
4. Gather one part and secure with a scrunchie and then also secure the other part.
5. Now divide the first section into two parts the same way. Start in the middle of your head and continue to the top of the ear.
6. Now your hair is divided in four distinct sections. Part each of these sections again, into two,three or four parts until you have manageable palm-sized sections. You should be able to keep the part in one hand while brushing or untangling with the other. A head usually makes 10 to 12 sections but it depends on the length and thickness of the strands. If the hair is less dense, four to eight sections may also do.

Moisturize
Before you start to untangle with any tool, make sure your hair is saturated with water and your favorite conditioner or detangler. You can use a spray bottle, but you can also do this while you are in the shower. Once you have some experience in untangling, the hair doesn't have to be completely wet, but your naps must always be flexible and supple to prevent breakage.

Untangle
Keep a section of hair in one hand and let your hand rest on the scalp. This prevents hair from pulling. Start combing or brushing at the ends with your other hand and work your way to the scalp. Make gentle plucking movements and don't try to pull through a snarl. Just stop, take the knot out by carefully separating strands with your hands and continue brushing or combing.

Untangle dry ends
If the ends of your hair feel a little dry, dip your comb or brush in pure Shea butter or coconut oil and start detangling the ends. Within no time, the brush should glide through and your ends will feel moisturized. Feel free to substitute Shea or coconut oil with your favorite detangler.

Washing hair

It is hard to say how often one needs to no-poo, but we need to wash hair on a regular basis to keep kinks and scalp clean. The frequency depends on the lifestyle as well as the hairstyle. Women who work out and those who wear their hair out will probably need to wash more frequently than others who don't work out and wear a lasting style like cornrows. However, no matter how durable the hairstyle, it should never be the only factor that determines the regularity of washing one's hair. Sebum and sweat are sterile, but the hair attracts dust and dirt from the polluted air and that needs to be washed out. The main deciding factor for washing should be whether the hair and scalp are unclean or not. If the hairstyle still looks good but the hair or scalp is unclean, do not wait, take the style out and wash the hair.

How to no-poo without knotting
The purpose of no-pooing is to clear one's hair and scalp from dust, sweat, pollution and product residue without stripping the strands of their natural moisture. Since our naps have the tendency to tangle, we have to be careful not stimulate knotting while no-pooing our hair. It can take hours to untangle kinky hair especially if it's longer than four inches. This routine will leave your hair clean without tangles and it will leave your hair feeling soft.

1. Divide the hair into six to 12 parts depending on the length and the thickness of your hair. Do not comb, just part the hair. If there is a knot, untangle with your fingers. Twirl or twist the part and tuck it in its base or use a clip to hold hair in place. Do this until all the hair is in tucked-in twirls.
2. Thoroughly wet the hair in the shower or under a tap. Make sure that hair is saturated.
3. Take a section out, loosen it and remove excess water. Add an ample amount of conditioner, saturate from root to end and massage the scalp. Twirl the section again and tuck it in once more.
4. Repeat until all the twirls are saturated and tucked in with conditioner.
5. Take the beginning twirl out and brush or comb the conditioner through with one of the gentle tools. Start at the ends and work up to the roots. After you finish, twirl the part and tuck in again.
6. Repeat until all the twirls are brushed through and tucked in.
7. Open the tap, let the water run through your tucked-in twirls. Take the initial twirl out. Let the water run through that part of the hair, rinsing the conditioner out. Don't comb, just let the water run through your coils. Once the conditioner is rinsed out, twirl and tuck in again.
8. Repeat until all the twirls are thoroughly rinsed out.

9. Pat hair to remove excess water and cover hair with an absorbent towel.

Tip: if you are not skilled enough and the twirls won't stay if you tuck them in, use hair clips. If you are very skilled and your hair is longer, you won't need a brush, you can untangle your hair with your fingers.

This method is very effective to clean the hair while leaving the naps soft. You can finish with the baking soda rinse described in the previous chapter. For a clarifying effect, add the juice of one large lemon to the amount of conditioner you normally use to wash your hair. This is as effective as any clarifying shampoo.

Hair that is shorter than four inch is easier to wash. You don't need to divide the hair in sections before you wash and you can start untangling after no-pooing. To wash hair:

1. Let the water run through your coils thoroughly wetting the hair.
2. Apply conditioner to the scalp and hair.
3. Start massaging the temples with your fingertips. Do not scrub. Gently move your fingertips in circular motions to the side, up the head and finally to the back of your head.
4. Use your fingers to distribute the conditioner through your hair. Don't disarrange the curls like we used to see in the commercials to create bubbles. Comb the conditioner through your hair with your fingers in one direction.
5. Allow the water to separate the coils and rinse the additional conditioner out of your hair.
6. Cover the hair with an absorbent towel. Do not rub the hair dry. Your hair should feel soft and ready to be styled. Untangle in sections while styling.

How to keep your scalp clean
Hair and scalp should always be kept clean, no matter the hairstyle. Even the most sophisticated, lasting hairstyle needs to be freshened after a while. Since washing the conventional way would disturb the hairstyle, we need to do this a different way. To keep the scalp fresh, you can use natural disinfectants like witch hazel. Use a cotton ball with a disinfectant of your choice to rub and clean the scalp in between the segments. Don't do this daily, and particularly not if you suffer from a dry scalp. The alcohol percentage is high in most of these formulas. Since alcohol has a drying effect, it can worsen your condition. Oiling your scalp afterwards can be a good way to prevent it from drying but be careful with this because some

oils are comedogenic - they clog pores. Use oil sparingly and use Jojoba or Tea Tree oil. Jojoba oil is an excellent oil to restore moisture and it will not clog the pores in the scalp. Tea Tree oil is a soothing and cleansing agent. After cleansing the scalp, the hair should also be refreshed. Mist the hairstyle with a natural spritz like the homemade Rosemary or Lavender and tie a scarf to absorb superficial dust and smooth the hair at the same time. This will also keep your hair moisturized.

Deep conditioning

Even if you no-poo frequently, a deep conditioning treatment on a regular basis is recommended. More so than a regular conditioner used for no-pooing, a deep conditioner can really boost the hair. Deep conditioners deeply penetrate the hair shafts, restoring and sealing in moisture and replacing valuable lost natural oils.

To deep condition:

1. Part the hair in manageable sections and saturate each section from root to end with deep conditioner.
2. Cover hair with a plastic cap and use a heating cap or a dryer to let the conditioner penetrate the hair. Read the instructions and don't exceed recommended time.
3. Thoroughly rinse the hair and pay attention to the hairline. Make sure there is no residue. Leftovers can harden hair strands and leave them fragile.
4. Cover hair with a clean, dry, absorbent towel. Hair is now ready to style as usual.

Hot oil treatments

Hot oil treatments are excellent for natural hair. They stimulate the scalp, add luster by restoring oils and enhance pliability of curls.

To do a hot oil treatment:

1. Part the hair in manageable sections.
2. To heat the oil, put it in a cup and place the cup in a bowl of hot water. You can also heat it in a microwave but be careful. Make sure the oil is not too hot. Test before you apply it on your hair.
3. Use a pastry brush to saturate a section of the hair with the heated oil from root to end. Use your hands or cotton balls if you don't have a pastry brush.
4. If you're done with a section, make a loose braid or twist, tuck it in and repeat for all sections. If this method doesn't hold, use clips.

5. Massage your scalp once all the sections are finished and cover head with a plastic cap for at least 45 minutes or overnight if possible.

6. *To wash hair after a hot oil treatment:*

7. Saturate each section one by one with your favorite no-poo conditioner before wetting the hair and tuck it back in.

8. Take the sections out one by one to thoroughly rinse them. Let the water run through the curls and finger comb to separate curls. Use a comb or brush if needed.

Dandruff and other scalp issues

Dandruff is a well-known scalp condition for many women of color who have used perms. It is, in fact, excessive shedding of the scalp and many of us are all too familiar with the gray-to-white flakes and irritated, itchy scalp. If you still suffer from dandruff after going natural, it is best to go and see a dermatologist to find out what the problem is. Very often, a dry and itchy scalp is mistaken for dandruff and a dermatologist can remedy your situation. A dry and itchy scalp could be the result of our hair care regimen. Hard water can irritate the scalp and so can poor scalp stimulation. Check the hardness level of your water, if this is ok, try different hair products. Ingredients in products can dry out or irritate the scalp. Being allergic to just one of the ingredients contained in a product can cause you to itch. Stop using shampoo and start no-pooing instead. Using natural hair products and remedies may also help eliminate your scalp issue.

Reducing temples and thinning spots

As long as your hair roots are not damaged, there is a chance that your temples and thinning spots will fill in. A dermatologist can determine whether your hair is permanently damaged or not. If your hair is not permanently damaged, there are products you can try to stimulate the follicles to grow. Even though, there is no guarantee that the product will work for you as well, it's best to go by word of mouth. New products become available everyday and it's hard to make a choice. Regularly check websites and ask around which products are worth trying. Always carefully follow the instructions of any product that you try and stop using it if you notice any unfavorable side effects.

A natural home remedy that might help is the homemade Rosemary spritz described in the "Natural nurturing" section. Daily spraying on the scalp's problem areas also seems to stimulate hair growth and fill in thinning spots.

Split ends

There are many theories about split ends but one thing is clear, they do not enhance the appearance of the hair. They make twists lay flat and the hair look lifeless. On top of that, they fuel tangles. You know that you have split ends when untangling seems like a never-ending task because the minute you untangle the kinks, they are not just tangling but really knotting again. If that is the case, your hair needs a trim.

The ends of your hair are another good indicator to verify if you have split ends. The ends of your naps will feel rough rather than smooth. A few split ends are harmless, but trimming hair is recommended if you have more than a few. It is hard to say how often or if one should trim at all to prevent split ends because not everyone develops split ends at the same rate and at the same speed. The best thing one can do is prevent frayed ends by tenderly taking care of the hair. Deep condition regularly, use the right tools and avoid using any kind of heat.

The golden rules for growing healthy hair

You will need patience to grow healthy, long, natural hair. Other than improving your diet, drinking plenty of water and exercise, and pursuing avenues that will improve your general health, there are not many things one can do to stimulate the hair growth process. Although certain vitamins or products may seem helpful for some people, there is no formula or product that guarantees hair growth for everyone. If you want to grow your hair healthy, be patient and follow these golden rules:

1. Tender hair needs tender care.
   Use a tender hand to care for your hair. Prevent your curls from tangling but also master the art of untangling.
2. When it comes to products, less is more.
   There is no need for a thousand different expensive products. Too many different products on one head only leave buildup and may clog pores.
   Look for a few basic products that work for your hair.
3. Tender hair needs gentle products and natural hair loves natural products.
   Stop using harsh shampoos and start reading product labels. Look for gentle and natural ingredients and products.
4. Keep hair and scalp clean.
   Regularly wash hair and scalp. Hair can only flourish on a scalp that is free from pollution, dust and product buildup.

5. Leave your hair alone.

This is key! Do you know why dreadlocks grow long? It is because hair is allowed to grow without being disturbed. Try to keep a hairstyle as long as possible but no longer than three months unless you want to loc your hair.

6. Moisture, moisture, moisture.

Water is your friend, so keep your curls moisturized all the time.

7. Say "no" to heat.

Avoid using heat appliances like blow dryers and stop using straightening irons altogether. They damage the coils and ruin the shape of your beautiful naps.

8. Trim your hair.

If you have split ends, trim your hair. Split ends tear up your strands and fuel tangling.

9. Enjoy your hair!

Transitioning; going natural gradually

Transitioning starts the minute the time has passed for your regular touch up. Unless one chooses to do the big chop before touch up time, everyone who has ever had her hair chemically treated will need to go through a period of transitioning to go natural. No beer rinse or any other product can reverse chemically altered hair to its natural texture. Relaxers and perms alter hair strands permanently so the only way to get rid of straightened parts of hair is to cut them.

During transitioning, your hair strands will carry two entirely different textures of hair: your natural kinky/curly texture that will be close to your scalp and the straightened ends. Hair can easily break at this point, the point where your naturally grown hair ends and the straightened part starts. This is called the point of demarcation. Handling straightened hair with naturally growing kinky roots is not easy because it has the tendency to tangle immensely which only stimulates breakages at the point of demarcation. While tangling of the two textures only gets worse as transitioning continues, the natural part of the hair will become softer and more manageable.

In the beginning, the natural part of the strands usually feels hard, crunchy and unmanageable. That is because the strands need time to heal. Straightening chemicals adversely affect hair and scalp and the new growth that initially comes out is what we call scab hair. This is hair that has been wounded by a relaxer or a perm. Hair roots are damaged the same way as when you are wounded by a relaxer and develop little burns. Like those burns, hair strands develop some scabbing as a protective reaction to the chemicals. This is what makes the new growth feels crunchy and unmanageable. Scabbing is also the reason many women end up in a vicious cycle of straightening. Many women are convinced that their natural hair is unmanageable and needs a relaxer to soften the strands. This is far from the truth. The chemicals may soften the strands temporarily, but they will probably only harden them more in the long run. It differs from person to person, but if you stop using the chemicals your hair will heal and return to its natural softness. It will literally be like scabs falling off. So don't panic if your hair feels dry and a little crunchy. The longer your natural hair grows the more your hair and scalp have a chance to heal. Some women experience a difference after the third month and some don't even experience scab hair at all.

Preparing to transition

If you feel more comfortable with longer hair and want your natural hair to have a certain length before doing the big chop, take your time to transition. The majority of women decide to transition before cutting off the relaxed ends.

The first two months of transitioning won't be difficult. You'll be able to wear your hair out without a problem but this will get harder in the fifth month or when the natural new growth exceeds two inches. Here are some tips if you decide on transitioning for a period longer than three months.

1. Set a deadline
   You are the only one who determines the period of transition and you decide when you want to cut the straightened ends. The deadline is only to have a sense of direction, and it is flexible. Most women do the big chop months before they reach the deadline date. Feel free to do so as well if you get tired of handling two textures. It hardly ever happens, but if you think your natural hair is not long enough by the time you've reached your deadline, feel free to extend as well.

2. Tangling
   Dealing with tangles is the hardest part of transitioning. Tangling is common during transitioning and the two different textures are the reason. Untangling your naturally kinky new growth will cause the straightened ends to tangle which is why sometimes you will have this idea of a never-ending untangling situation. One way to ease untangling is to dip a nappy-friendly hair brush in Shea butter or your favorite detangler and start untangling the ends and work your way to the scalp. Always take your time to untangle if you want to keep your length. Impatience and pulling will lead to knots and breakage. Mastering the art of untangling described in Chapter 4 might also be helpful while you're transitioning.

3. Breakage
   Prepare yourself for some breakage. One can hardly avoid breakage during transitioning. Hair is likely to break at the line of demarcation during untangling. Also expect the ends to break because they are the oldest part of the hair. As the oldest part of the strands, the ends, are also prone to breakage because they have had the most to endure and it is very likely that they will be brittle.

4. Trim your ends regularly
   Split ends and brittle ends promote excessive tangling. Clipping your ends on a regular basis will save you split ends and therefore some tangling and breakage as well. Dealing with two textures is hard enough.

5. Braids, twists and other lasting styles
   If you want to transition for a period longer than six months, braids and other lasting styles are your best choice. Afrikan hair grows best when left undisturbed so keep your hair in lasting styles as much as possible so that you don't have to untangle on a daily basis.

Transition styles and care

Relaxed hair requires different hair care than natural hair, so you will need to combine the two different hair care methods. Keep using your favorite products in the beginning but also start looking for products for natural hair in the meantime. If your new growth is half an inch or longer, try pure Shea butter, coconut oil or other moisturizers designed or recommended for natural hair. This is a way to find out which products you like and work for your natural hair. If your hair gains length, it is up to you to if you also want to use the same product for the straightened ends. It all about what you like and what your hair prefers. Since you will still use several different products weekly, no-pooing is recommended to regularly get rid of residue. Weekly deep conditioning treatments are recommended as well because they can help strengthen the hair strands and make them more manageable and that is very necessary with the two textures.

The first three to six months of transitioning, you will be able to wear your hair out without a problem. To prepare yourself for the look of natural hair you may want to wear curly hairstyles like twists, twist-out and straw-sets. Not only are these styles good to prepare oneself for the new natural look, they look good and it is a way to avoid heat from blow dryers and curling irons.

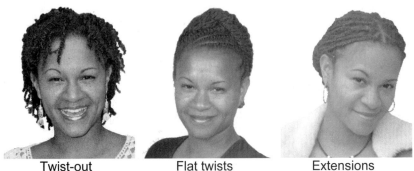

| Twist-out | Flat twists | Extensions |

Figure 6. Transitioning styles

Twist-out

Condition wash and towel dry. Use pure Shea butter or another moisturizer designed for natural hair to soften your new growth if it is half an inch or longer. Start parting your hair like you would if you would do a roller set. Make two-strand twist of the sections instead. If the twists won't stay in, use curling paper or a curling rod to secure the ends. Let hair air dry and take out when the hair is completely dry. Finger comb hair to style.

Braid-out

Same as twist-out but make braids instead of twists.

Straw set

You will need: Straws, Bobby pins and setting lotion

Condition, wash and towel dry. Cut the straws to the size that is about the width of the rollers that used to roller set your straightened hair. Start parting your hair. Make sure that the section is not wider than the cut straw. Smooth the hair use a setting lotion of your choice and roll the ends around the straw. Take out the straws if hair is completely dry. Shake your head to loosen the curls and use your fingers to style but do not comb. The style will last until the next wash. Meanwhile keep scalp clean and oil as needed.

Curling paper

Use curling paper instead of regular rollers to curl your hair. This is also a way to prepare yourself for your natural look.

Protective hairstyles
After six months, or when your new growth has reached three inches depending on your hair growth speed, it will become more difficult to blend the two textures and untangling will also become very hard. From this point on, braids and protective styles that you can wear for at least a week in a row are your best choices. This avoids untangling and breakage on a daily basis. Combination styles where the front is cornrowed or flat-twisted are a good choice because they camouflage the difference in texture, the ends are protected and most of these styles can last for a week or two. By this time, your natural hair growth is probably thick and healthy, so it might also be a good time to try extensions. These are lasting styles that can give your hair a long break from untangling hassles and also totally hide the texture difference.

Emergencies
Not everyone's hair is strong enough to keep two textures. Some women have to deal with excessive breakage while transitioning. Breakage will appear at the point of demarcation and the new natural growth will show through thin relaxed hair. The best thing one can do in this case is the big chop. If you don't feel comfortable with short hair, transition with extensions or a weave because the breakage will only get worse.

The Big Chop (BC)

The big chop is the most significant step of the natural journey or the most vigorous way to start it. It is the realization of the transformation from relaxed to natural hair. This transformation becomes reality when one cuts off the chemically altered part of the strands so that the hair is completely natural. It is a big step for most women because many of us are attached to length. Women don't like to cut their hair and a short natural is not a hairstyle that many women of color desire. This is not the only reason why the big chop is a big step. Another reason is the fear of the unknown. For most, the big chop is scary because they don't know what to do with their natural hair. In spite of suffering from hair breakage and other inconveniences, at least women of color know how to handle straightened hair. To have to deal with natural hair, all of a sudden, could be intimidating, particularly after a lifetime of straightening. The image that nappy hair is impossible to handle and needs to be fixed does not make the big chop any more appealing either.

Clearly doing the big chop doesn't only signify a physical change but also a mental one. Someone who is ready to do the big chop and who is prepared to care for their natural hair has overcome prejudices, misconceptions and mental barriers. These are huge accomplishments in a natural journey.

While some gradually have to overcome all the hurdles step by step and hesitate to do the big chop, others have no problem doing it right away. They start the journey with freshly cut natural hair. Since the variety of short-cropped natural styles, this group of "big choppers" who used to be a minority, is currently the fastest growing group.

In the center of those who immediately chop, and those who postpone the big chop, is the largest group. This group gets used to the idea of the big chop fairly easy and does it after a couple of months of transitioning. Fact of the matter is that everyone who is going natural has to chop eventually. There is no better time to do it than when one is ready. And again, you are the best judge when it comes to your own hair. You will know when you are ready to do the big chop.

Preparing for the BC

When you are ready for the big chop, you may want to go to a barber instead of a salon. It can be somewhat difficult to find a nappy-friendly salon or one that specializes in natural hair. Barbers have a life long experience of shaping and cutting afro styles, so you should be in good hands. Another advantage is that most barbers are cheaper than salons. If you don't know a barber, ask around. If you see a Black man or woman with well-shaped or trimmed hair, ask the person for information about the place he or she had his or her hair done.

Think about how you want your hair before doing the big chop. Do you want your hair shaped? What kind of shape would you like your hair to be? Or, do you want your 'fro to be shaped at all? The options are numerous, even for a teeny weeny afro, also called TWA. Some people like a round shape, others like a fade, etc. Some just want the relaxed ends cut out and do not care about a shape, because they want twists and are ready to experiment. It all depends on what you like. You'd be well advised to think about it before going to the barber's so that you don't have to make a decision on the spot.

Wash, untangle and moisturize the night before visiting the barber. Before cutting your hair, the barber has to comb through your hair. This is no fun if your hair is tangled and dry. Take this opportunity to say farewell to your chemically altered tresses. It will be the last time you will comb through your hair with permed ends, so say goodbye while no-pooing, moisturizing and untangling. Sing a song, dance or think of some ritual for a dignified farewell. Say goodbye to the high maintenance, permed hair era and open up to discover the stress-free maintenance of natural hair.

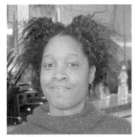 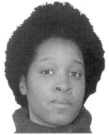 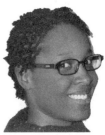

| Before the BC | After the BC | End Style |

Figure 7. The Big Chop

Advantages of the BC

Apart from starting fresh, the big chop has two other advantages. If you cut off all permed hair, you can focus on your own newly discovered hair. This is a wonderful advantage. There is no distraction of relentless breakage and tangling or trying to conceal either the straightened hair or the curly part. You can immediately discover your own hair's beauty all over again. You will learn to appreciate your unique textures of hair and find out what works best for your naps. You can spend time trying great styles with your freshly cut natural hair. While doing all of this, you and your naps can grow old and long together.

Versatility

Another big advantage of the big chop is versatility. Short naturals are more versatile than ever. Besides the old TWA you can try Comb Coils, Twists, Twist-Outs, Bantu knots, small braids, tucked-in-braids, and Cornrows just to name a few. All these hairstyles can be done with as little as two inches of natural Afrikan hair and it's a very good idea to try some of them. Not only is it a lot of fun, they are also very chic and versatile. And, although it might seem unbelievable now, soon enough your hair will be too long to wear these styles as chic as they are when your hair is still short.

Natural styles and care

TWA's

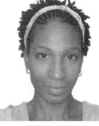

Even the TWA has enough versatility not to get boring. You can wear the nice round-shaped 'fro, free form 'fro, chunky 'fro or one of those out-fro styles; twist, braids or coils out. Taking care of a short, natural one is the easiest of all regimens. It's either get up and go or no-poo and go.

Figure 8. TWA style: flat twists in the front, two strand twists in the back.

TWA styles
First, enjoy your freshly cut hair. Feel how soft your naps are. Take a good look at those beautiful ringlets of coils. They are yours and you will be able to do more things with your natural naps than you have ever imagined. Knowing how to care for your naps is key. Take your time. Remember, Rome wasn't built in one day either.

Free form 'fro
No-poo or rinse and pat dry. Style your hair by coiling the ends of your curls randomly. If you don't like to wet your hair in the shower, spray your hair with one of those spritzes mentioned in the previous section addressing products. If you want more length, braid the hair at night in chunks, do not comb. Take the braids out in the morning, coil, shape and go.

Plopping
If you have the type of hair that has well-defined curls when it's wet but curls that become frizzy when you pat them dry, plopping might be something for you. It's a way to keep the curls defined and the frizz down if you want to wear your hair out. Rather than walking around with dripping wet hair, wrap your soaking wet hair in a towel or t-shirt after a shower. Keep your hair wrapped for about 10 minutes to have the excessive water absorbed and let the natural shape of curls set. If you need products to enhance the curls' shape, add them while your hair is still soaking wet before you wrap the hair.

Twist-out 'fro
Depending on the size of the twists, this could be a curly or a chunky 'fro. The smaller the twists, the curlier the afro.

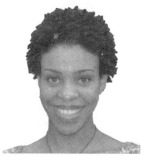

How to
Mist and twist hair before going to bed. Take twists out in the morning, shape, style and go.

Braid-out 'fro
The only difference with the twist-out 'fro is that you make braids instead of twists. And, the result is completely different. A braid-out 'fro is more like a stretched or blowout afro.

Figure 9. Coiled twist out 'fro

How to
Braid the hair at night and take them out in the morning. Don't comb hair, but just shape, style and go.

Shaped 'fro
First, your barber has to shape your 'fro the way you want it. To keep it in model daily, you can no-poo or rinse, pick while hair is still moist, shape and go. Mind you, your 'fro will shrink while drying. If you want a more fluffy, stretched looking 'fro, make some braids before going to bed. Carefully take the braids out and style with your hands and fingers. Only pick if necessary, shape and go. If you want a perfect shaped 'fro use a silky or satin scarf. Cover your 'fro with the scarf and carefully slide it off after a couple of seconds.

Afro puff
The puff is an afro is pulled back together with a head band. It is a favorite afro style for many new naturals.

How to
This popular hairstyle is very easy to do. Whether your hair is wet or dry you can always make a puff. You only need a headband or a scarf. Just place the headband on your hairline, then slowly pull the hair back and secure the band.

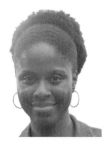

Figure 10. Afro puff

Afro care
Whether you wear a shaped 'fro or any kind of 'fro that doesn't require combing, try to condition your hair biweekly. After 10 days of wearing your hair loose without combing, hair will probably start matting and locing, thereby making it difficult to untangle your hair. This is so even if it feels soft. Unless you want your hair loced, deep condition your hair after seven to 10 days and untangle your hair. Don't just comb. No-poo the way described in the previous chapter.

Coils

Coils are an ideal change for any length of natural hair from a TWA to long hair. Coils can be styled with as little as one inch of hair and there is no limit to the length that can keep a coil.

How to do coils

~ No-poo hair and towel dry. Hair should be at least somewhat damp before coiling so keep a spritz bottle at hand in case hair does begin to dry.

~ Part hair in pencil size section and add your favorite moisturizer or oil to the section. Some people like to use a clear, alcohol-free gel, but this is optional.

~ Place thumb and index finger at the root of the hair, near the scalp. Roll the section between thumb and forefinger and roll hair clockwise around index finger - the way you would curl your hair around your finger.

~ Keep twirling as hair begins to coil. Slowly slide down when the coil becomes tight until you reach the end of hair.

Coil Care
Coils will look nice for one to two weeks or until the next wash. Do not keep this style longer than three weeks. The more products you need for a style, the less time you are able to keep the style. Scalp may itch due to commercial product use as well as from the attraction of dust. Keep scalp clean with Witch Hazel, spritzes and natural oils.
The coils can easily be taken out by twirling them in opposite directions.

Coil out variant
Try a coil out for a change. Carefully separate the coils for a coil-out and finger comb.

Twists

Twists are a most versatile hairstyle. You can create updos or wear them loose. Twists are just two strands of hair that are wound around each other. Our different Afrikan textures naturally create a rope-like and curly effect.
The easiest way to learn twists is to have it done by a friend or at a salon and re-twist it yourself after a week or two.

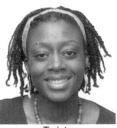 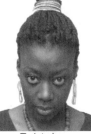 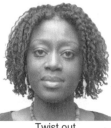

Twists   Twists bun   Twist out

Figure 11. Versatality of twists

Take the twists down
Start at the base of the twist, near your scalp, put your index finger in the middle of the twist and pull your finger down. If you get stuck, start loosening the end of the twist up to the point where you were stuck.

To re-twist

It's best to re-twist hair after washing. The hair doesn't have to be wet as long as it is fresh and clean.

~ Unravel both strands completely to prevent the hair from locing and to remove possible lint.

~ Add your favorite moisturizer. Use a spray bottle to moisten the hair if it's very dry.

~ Brush or comb the section.

~ Divide the section in two equal strands.

~ Twist one strand around the other in a twisting motion until the end.

~ Moisten your fingers with water or your favorite moisturizer and twirl the ends of the twist around your fingers to give it a natural curl.

Pay attention to the ends, they give the style a neat finished look. If the ends are bluntly cut, they will tend to unravel. In this case, use curling paper or a small roller to secure and curl the twist. If the ends feel rough and don't give the twists that naturally curly end, it's probably time for a trim.

Quick and easy
Twisting hair is not that difficult but it can be overwhelming to do your own hair. The smaller the twists, the more time it will take to finish the hairstyle but you should know that you don't have to spend a whole day twisting. You can spread it over a couple of days, even weeks, while wearing slightly different hairstyles. The idea is to break it down in manageable pieces and to go from big or medium to small twists. Here is the routine for quick and easy twists.

~ No-poo and pat dry.
Twists done on wet or damp hair tend to shrink. but after a couple of days. they will loosen naturally. If you just want loose twists with some length, let your hair dry before twisting.

~ Part your hair in four sections like described in the previous chapter in the paragraph "The art of untangling."

~ Now loosen one section, divide it in four parts and twist each part.

~ Repeat for the three other sections.

Your hair will be in 16 twists. If you think they are too big continue, divide each twist in two again, so you'll have 32 twists. You can continue doing this depending on your time and the style you desire. You can wear 16 or 32 twists for one week and then divide each twist in two so you'll have a new hairstyle with smaller sections.

Twist care
Twists are easy to maintain and they can last up to four weeks. You can no-poo them, rinse them and spray them. It all depends on your preference. Tie the hair before going to bed to prevent frizzy twists and oil the scalp as needed. Frizzy looking twists can be re-twisted by using some water and moisturizer.

Twist-out
This crimpy hairstyle is the most favorite after the twists. This style normally lasts for a couple of days but you can wear a full head of these fabulous crimps for a week if you know the secret to it. The tricks to extend the lifetime of a twist-out are:

One day before wearing the twist-out

~ Rinse the twists and saturate the twists with the homemade natural styling spray or use another styling aid that can hold the crimps.

~ Re-twist the ones that are a bit loose. The firmer the twists the longer the crinkles will last.

~ Pin the twists out of your face or in a model you prefer.

~ Let the hair completely dry, preferably by air drying.

The day of the twist-out and the days after

~ Carefully take the twists out. Start at the base of the twist, near your scalp. Put your index finger between of the strands of the twist while unwinding and pull your finger down. If you get stuck, start loosening the end of the twist up to the point where you were stuck.

~ Do not comb the hair for as long as you want to wear you the twist-out; use your fingers to style.

~ Tie the hair before going to sleep and oil the scalp as needed.

Bantu knots

Bantu knots are so versatile, they are ideal for a chic night out as well as for a hot summer day on the beach. They complement the features of a face and place an emphasis on beautiful eyes.

As with the twists, the easiest way to learn to do bantus is to have the style done for you and then re-do it yourself.

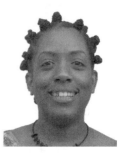

Figure 12. Bantu knots

How to do Bantus

- No-poo hair and towel dry.
- Part hair in sections and add your favorite moisturizer or oil and an alcohol-free gel to the section.

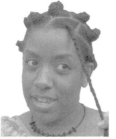

- Make a twist, braid, or coil - Bantus can be started with any one.
- Hold your coil, twist or braid at its base close to the scalp.
- Use your wise finger to keep the coil, twist or braid at its base while wrapping the rest of it around its base.

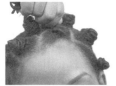
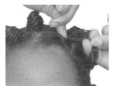
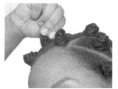

Hold your coil, twist or braid at its base	Hold the Bantu-to-be at its base	Wrap around the base until the you reach the end

Figure 13 How to do Bantu Knots

Normally our hair texture keeps a Bantu knot in place but feel free to use a hairpin to secure the knot if it does not hold.

Bantu care

If you wear Bantu knots, twists or braids, try to wear them for at least one complete week; the longer the better but not for longer than four weeks.

Keep your scalp clean with Witch Hazel and natural oils like jojoba and tea tree oil. Keep hair moist and fresh with homemade spritzes.

Take out Bantus:
Find the end of the Bantu, wind it to the opposite direction to loosen it. If the Bantu style was based on coils, uncoil hair by twirling into the opposite direction. If the style was based on twist, untwist the hair, starting at the beginning of the twist. If you do this with all the bantus you will have a coily style. You can wear this style for a couple of days. Pamper your hair with a honey-olive oil treatment before you take the style out.

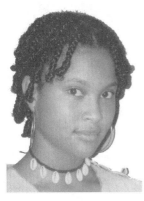

Figure 14. Contemporary braids

Braids
Braids are the most common hairstyle in Afrikan hair care. That is hardly a surprise. They have always been part of our cultural life and can be traced back as far as 2630 B.C. in the Third Dynasty of the ruler Akhethoptep in Egypt. In those days, braids represented more than just a hairstyle. They were integrated in cultural and ceremonial life and could announce a pregnancy or signify a social or a marital status. The appreciation of braids declined when the hairstyles of captive Afrikans were projected as offensive by the western world. In some states, women were obliged by law to cover their heads in public.

As a consequence, the stigmatized braids were demoted to hairstyles to wear at home or under a wig but not for the outside world to see. The cultural revolution of the 1960's laid the foundation for the braids to make a comeback. Now they are as popular as ever and it's hard to believe that it took a couple of lawsuits in the 1980s before braids were accepted in corporate life.The many various braid styles we see today can truly be called Afrikan-American hairstyles because they genuinely represent a mixture of two continent's cultures. Braids are easy to do and easy to maintain. Many braided styles can be completed in one hour, and more often than not, the style will last for at least one week. These styles can be easily maintained by tying the hair with a scarf at night.

Cornrows

Cornrows are braids that are intertwined to lie flatly on the scalp. This is a typical Afrikan-American name and they are probably named after the similarity of orderly rows of corn on the cob.

Cornrows offer infinite hairstyling. Styles vary from classic and chic to professional and simple everyday styles. Not only can you choose between numerous hairstyles, but there is also diversity in the way the cornrows themselves are braided. The rows can vary from small to thick or large and very often extensions are used these days to extend the lifetime of a style and to make the rows look fuller. There is also a difference in the way the extensions are intertwined. This is particularly noticeable at the

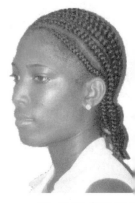

Figure 15. Cornrow

front. Some hairstylist start subtly and leave a bit of your own hair before intertwining extensions while others start doing this from the very beginning of a cornrow.

Another choice would be whether you like the rows braided very closely together without the scalp being exposed or not so closely together and have the scalp exposed. Cornrows that are braided so closely together that they completely cover the scalp without the parting being exposed are called knitrows.

Some pleasant advantages of wearing cornrows is that it's an enduring and easy to care for hairstyle. Most styles last for at least two weeks so your hair can rest from manipulation and pulling and the only maintenance that is necessary to keep cornrows neat is tying up a scarf before going to bed. The scalp should also be cleaned regularly if the style will carry over for longer than one week.

The only disadvantage of this style is that it could be inconvenient while being braided as it is done flatly on the scalp. A little inconvenience is ok but a hairstyle should never be braided so tight that it hurts. If this is the case, take the style out. Tight braiding will only harm your strands.

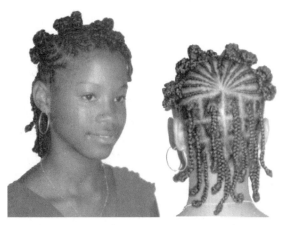

Figure 16. A combination of cornrows, single braids and bantus.

Flat twists and Silky twists

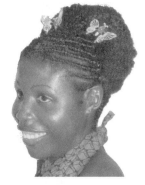

Flat twists are two stranded twists that are intertwined flatly on the scalp. They look like cornrows and they are at least as versatile but they have a slightly softer look. Naturally flat twist styles last for two to three weeks and, as with cornrows, little maintenance is required. Tying up the hair at night is all that is required to keep the style neat. When the hair is a little frizzy, you can refresh the style by misting it with a homemade spray and then tie the head for about 10 minutes. The scalp should be cleaned every three to four days and oiled as needed.

Figure 17. Flat twist updo

Silky twists are like flat twists but instead of twists coils are intertwined flatly on the scalp. In fact, the hair is smoothly rolled to the scalp using oil and gel to create a silky look. The maintenance is no different from that of flat twists. Synthetic hair can be used for both types of twists to give a style more body and hold. Extensions usually extend the lifetime of the hairstyle but the maintenance is the same as when it's done with one's natural hair.

Banding

Banding is a century-old technique that was popular to create sculpture-like hairstyles. Today, the same method is used to make distinguished or playful hairstyles and also to stretch natural hair. We speak of banding when ribbons or bands are wrapped around sections of hair. Taking out the bands of hair that have been allowed to dry completely will give natural hair a longer look almost like when the hair has been blown-out effect.

Banding gained popularity because it safer than the use of heat appliances. As long as you make sure that you don't use rubber bands or other types of bands made from material that is harmful to the kinks, banding is safe. Other than that, the same rules apply as for braids; don't band too tightly and don't leave them in for a period longer than three months.

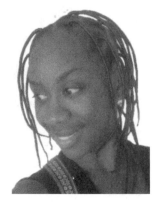

Figure 18. Banding

Going locs

Locs are the most natural way to grow long Afrikan hair. Since the coils that appear in natural hair have the tendency to group together, nappy hair will naturally bond together after a period of being undisturbed. This is how locs begin to form. Gathered kinks and coils will loc if not being combed or brushed for months in a row. No chemicals or additional hair products are necessary. Your hair will do the job just by being left alone. That doesn't mean you can grow locs overnight. It takes time, patience and care to grow and maintain well-groomed locs. It is a commitment but one look at some beautiful locs you occasionally spot and you know it is worth the effort.

Starting yourself or by a professional

Even if you want to take care of your locs yourself, it is recommend to start your locs by a professional or someone with experience. This is important because the way your hair is parted and the size of the sections will determine the look of your future dreadlocks. If you are not satisfied when your hair begins to loc, you will need to take them down and start all over again. Dividing hair into sections that are too small may also cause locs to break when locs grow longer. An experienced person will know what size is right for your hair texture and your volume of hair and will be able to advice you. If you insist on starting them yourself, play it safe and take pencil size sections. Sections of this size normally provide a strong enough base for a locs so that it won't break.

Get a clean start

Locks should always be started with freshly washed, clean hair. The hair should be very clean without any debris or residue of a conditioner or other hair products. Debris and residue will make your locs look dull if they loc into your hair. That is why shampooing is recommended when starting locs. Use a pH-balanced or an herbal shampoo.

Hair should be damp when starting locs so that the hair can easily be shaped into the desired style. Use clips to keep hair in place, never use force. Keep a spray bottle at hand to keep hair moist in case the hair dries while working on the locs-to-be.

No beeswax, butters or petroleum based products

Never ever start locs with beeswax or similar products. These products will keep your hair together initially but it will be almost impossible to get the stuff out of your hair.

Aloe Vera is excellent for locing

Aloe Vera is excellent for locing. The natural gel nourishes the hair and stimulates kinks to loc. You can use pure Aloe Vera out of a bottle from the health store or make your own. If you make your own gel, scoop out the gel and make sure that there is absolutely nothing but colorless liquid. Use a coffee filter to sieve the green plant pieces from the residue. You don't want any kind of residue loced into your hair.

Time to loc

Depending on your hair type it will take anywhere from eight months to one year before hair is truly loced. The tighter the curl, the easier hair will loc. Wavy or straight hair may take as long as one and a half years to two years to loc.

Starting loc techniques

Locs can be started in many different ways. The most common way is to start locs with palm rolls, comb coils, twists or braids. Since dreadlocks became fashionable, old techniques are being revived and new methods have been developed. Back combing is one of the old techniques with a new name while Nu locs, Sisterlocks™, Riqui locs and Twisty locs are newly developed salon methods to start dreadlocks.

Think about the kind of locs you want before starting them. Do you want big or small locs, do you want free form or cultivated locs. Your choice to select one of these methods should not only be determined by your hair type and your hair length but also, if not primarily, by your convenience.

Starting locs with coils or palm rolls

Hair type: Tight and medium O
Hair Length: One inch and up
Advantage: looks smooth
Coils and rolls are a most common way to start locs. The little kinks in tight to medium type-O curls, keep a strand together and cause them to loc naturally. If you want to start small, smooth looking locs coils or palm rolls should be your choice depending on the length of your hair. Start with comb coils if your hair is short, one to three inches, start with palm rolls if your hair is longer.

Disadvantage: high maintenance, takes a long time before hair locs
Comb coils and palm rolls are the most challenging way to start locs because they don't hold very well and easily frizz in a humid environment. These styles last until the next wash. Water will cause coils and rolls to unravel which is why it will take much longer for hair to locs. Frequent grooming is also required to keep the coils shaped; at least once every two weeks and certainly after every wash.

Starting locs with two-strand twists
Hair types: All
Hair Length: Two inches
Advantages: Looks like a loc from the start, inexpensive
Twists are an ideal way to start locs for most kinky hair types. They enhance the curly structure of nappy hair while looking like locs from the start. The kinky curls bind the hair together naturally which is an advantage during the process of locing.

Disadvantage: Frizziness
Frequent grooming may be necessary to keep your hair looking neat if your hair easily frizzes. This will depend on your hair type as well as the environment you live in because twists tend to get frizzy in humid weather. They can also unravel and unwind when hair growing or during washing if the hair is short or of the looser type S. In this case frequent grooming will be required but be careful and don't over twist the hair. Too much twisting will damage the hair and will cause breakage.

There are two ways of using twists as a basis to start locs. The most common way is to let the two strands grow to be one loc. The second way is to separate and re-twist the hair until the single strands are fully locked. It takes a little more maintenance, and it will take longer before the individual stands mash together, but this way one can grow thinner locs.

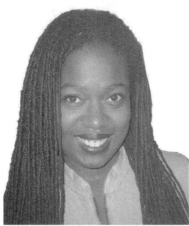
Dreadlocks started with braids

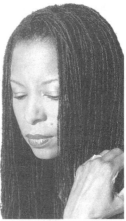
Sisterlocks™

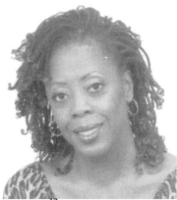
Spicy locs[17] started with twists

Figure 19. Different kinds of locs

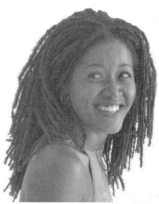
Locks started with coils

Starting locs with Senegalese Twists
Hair types: All
Hair Length: Three inches and up
Advantage: Low maintenance
An easier way to grow locs based on coils is to start out with Senegalese twists. These are two-strand twists but the strands are coiled before they are twisted. The twisted coils hold much better than single coils; they last after washing and frizz less. Thus, less maintenance and hardly any grooming will be required to grow locs. The strands will start locing individually as coils before they will loc together as a Senegalese twist. So if you keep separating and re-twisting the style, you will have thin coiled locs in the end.

Disadvantage: Skilled hairdresser needed
Since the Senegalese twists is not a common style, you may need a skilled hairdresser to start and maintain the locs. This is important because the hair needs to be twisted in one direction. Twisting the hair in different directions will work against the locing process and may cause the hair to break.

Starting locs with braids
Hair type: All
Hair Length: long enough to keep a braid; two inches and up
Advantage: durability, less grooming
Braids are ideal to start locs if it is difficult for one's hair to hold a twist or a coil. This method is also ideal if you want to start locs quickly without a lot of maintenance. Braids keep hair strands together rather tightly allowing hair to locs fast with hardly any frizz. Washing hair may cause a little frizzier braids but that's all. They won't unwind so you won't have to wait two weeks before the first wash.

Disadvantage: scalp exposure
The only disadvantage is that a little more scalp will be exposed in the beginning when the style is fresh because braids are tighter in stitch than coils or twists. This will end quickly as the hair begins to grow.

Sisterlocks™
Hair type: All
Hair Length: One and a half inches of new growth and up
Advantage: very thin locs, no need to cut off relaxed part
Sisterlocks™ is a locing method developed by Dr. JoAnne Cornwell designed to create a new style based on the unique texture of Afrikan hair. The locs are thinner than the usual ones so they allow more flexibility than

the common, thicker locs. Most typical about this technique is that you can keep your length; you don't have to do the big chop to start these locs. Sisterlocks™ can be done with one and a half inches of new growth and the straightened ends can be cut off over time.

Another advantage is that, like with the braids-method, Sisterlocks™, the hair strands keep well together allowing hair to loc fast with hardly any frizz because the locs are created according to one's texture. A certified consultant will instruct you how to wash your hair until the locs are set but the locs-to-be won't unwind easily so you won't have to wait for weeks before the first wash.

Disadvantage: Dependency
The main drawback is that you need a certified consultant trained by the proficiency standards of Sisterlocks™ . This is costly and you will be dependent until your hair is fully loced and you learn how to maintain the style yourself.

Twisty Locs
Hair type: All, relaxed
Hair Length: Two inches of new growth
Advantage: micro locs, no need to cut off relaxed part
Twisty locs are the thinnest kind of cultivated locs; they are, in fact, micro locs. An interlocking technique is used create the locs to look like a very thin twists. Like Sisterlocks™, these micro locs stay well into the hair and you don't have to cut off the relaxed part of your hair to start these locs. The difference is that you will need two inches of new growth instead of only one and a half.

Disadvantage: Expensive, dependency
This method is quite expensive. You can only get price information after a consultation and the price will be based on the length and the condition of your hair. Only a trained hairdresser can twisty loc your hair and maintain the style. This is a disadvantage because you will be dependent on a hairdresser for maintenance.

Riqui Locs
Hair type: All
Hair Length: One and a half inches
Advantage: thin locs, low maintenance
Riqui locs is a new way of locing which was developed by hairstylist Richelle Braithwaite who resides in Brooklyn. Like the braids-method, Riqui Locs keep the hair strands well together allowing hair to loc with hardly any

frizz. This is a rather easy way to start locs because maintenance is only recommended when one feels the need for this and one can also be taught how to maintain the style.

Disadvantage: Limited to the Brooklyn area
The drawback is that this is a fairly new method that is being patented, so until then, only Riqui herself can do your iocs.

Starting locs with extension: Yarn locs, Silky locs, locs Fusion
Hair type: All, also relaxed hair
Hair length: One inch and up
Pros: immediate length, almost care-free
Locs with extensions are another opportunity to start locs for hair that is difficult to loc - relaxed hair or naturally straight, wavy hair. If you are too impatient to grow lengthy locs or you don't want to cut off your relaxed hair extension, locs are an option to consider. After your own hair is coiled, twisted or braided an extension is attached to or wrapped around it. The difference in Yarn, Silky and Fusion is the extension material used. Yarn gives locs a kind of matte finish, Silky locs have a smooth and shiny finish, while a more afro hair type of extension is used for locs Fusion giving locs a more matte and natural look. Make sure you are well informed before choosing any type of extension. Some extensions, like wool, take very long to dry and some may dry out your hair.

Cons: requires professional care
Not only do you need a professional to put the locs in for you, will also need a professional to keep your hair healthy and clean. Wearing extensions cause lint at the root between extension and hair. A loctician[ξ] familiar with this method should be able to prevent debris from locking in your hair. Depending on the method used, the extension locs will be cut out of your hair or taken out.

Free-form locs vs. organic locs
The term, free-form refers to locs that are being formed to themselves when one stops to comb the hair. Hair will start to mesh and loc irregularly. Free form locs are the most carefree style among locs because these locs do not require re-twisting, palm rolling or tightening of the roots. Freeformers only separate their locs. This doesn't mean that the hair is not kept clean. The irregularly formed clusters of hair should also be washed and kept free of lint.

[ξ] See glossary

Free form locs can be started several ways. One popular way is to towel dry freshly washed hair in circular motions and let the locs be formed by coils. Never comb or brush hair and wash as often as you wish. Another way is to start with a twist-out and separate coiled clusters when hair starts to mesh. Some people also start with twists or coils and then simply stop shaping locs. They let the hair do its own thing without re-twisting or palm rolling.

Organic locs are different from free-form locs in that there is no predetermined style. There is also no shaping, nor separating of locs. Hair locs into one or several big clusters. This is a rather carefree hair style as well, but again, keeping hair clean of lint is also a must.

Loc stages

Before your locs establish, they will go through three different stages; the baby phase, the teenage phase and the mature phase. Depending on your hair texture, it will take one to one and a half years to be completely loced. While you're in the loc process, there is only one constant factor: your hair is growing.

Baby phase

At the beginning in this baby phase, hair should be handled very carefully. The focus will be on keeping the hair from unraveling to allow the locs to settle. This period lasts about three to six months, depending on your hair texture and the method you choose. The locs-to-be will puff up at first, lose their smooth, glossy look and start to frizz. After a couple of weeks, hair will shrink because the coils are starting interlock and form buds randomly. Buds are little knots in the middle or at the end of the loc-to-be. This is an indication that locs are starting to settle. It is comparable to the buds of flowers; the buds will also allow your locs bloom over time.

Grooming

Most locticians will recommend not washing the hair with water for at least two weeks when starting locs with twists or even three to four weeks when starting with palm rolls or coils. The reason for this is that wetting the hair will loosen up the locs-to-be and it's best to leave the hair undisturbed to allow the locs to settle.

Keep your scalp clean at all times and immediately remove dust or lint from your hair in this stage. Once lint locs into your hair, it is very difficult to take out. If you can't stand not washing your hair for so long, just go ahead and wash it. The only disadvantage is that it will take some more maintenance and a bit longer for the locs to settle. Braids, Sisterlocks and extension locs can be washed as usual. Always wash the locs carefully in the baby phase. Massage the scalp gently and try not to disturb the loc-sections.

Maintenance

To shape up your locs-to-be, wrap the loose and frizzy hairs around the nearest loc-section and clip them securely. This is called re-twisting or simply twisting. Do this after your hair is freshly washed and still damp. Twisting hair dry may cause damage because of the friction which can lead to thin, fragile locs which will eventually break. You can use pure Aloe Vera or some natural oil like avocado, coconut or olive oil to help keep the hair in place. Use oils sparingly and always wrap hair in the same direction around the twist. Re-twisting locs in different directions can also cause locs to break. Be aware that nappy hair does not shine; it absorbs light rather than reflect it. If you think your hair looks dull, do a hot oil treatment before shampooing or use just a little oil to re-twist the strands. Use clips to keep hair in place then let the hair air dry or use a hooded dryer at medium heat.

The baby stage can be challenging. Some parts will look frizzy and other parts may unwind. This is especially so if you started with coils, palm rolls or twists. It has to do with the different textures of hair on one's head, as some textures interlock easier than other ones. Your commitment will be tested if you care for your locs yourself. New growth tends to unwind a minute after it is re-twisted. This is all part of the loc journey. Don't keep twisting and try to shape your hair in this phase. Over twisting will cause hair to weaken and thin at the roots, which will lead to breakage. If it's really too much to handle, consult a loctician.

Sleeping with a satin of silky cap will help minimize frizz.

Teenage phase

This is the stage where you will notice your locs lengthening. The locs are already settled but not completely established yet. This phase can last anywhere from three months to one year. There is more budding and the buds actually start to loc. Locs will still be frizzy and growth that goes along with frizziness could be perceived as hair going wild because it does not "behave" like you expect.

In this stage, locs also tend to lock to each other. This is called crawling. It happens when strands of a particular loc creep to a neighboring loc. Do not worry, much like teenagers, your locs only need some attention and guidance to become independent, mature locs. Crawling locs simply need to be popped. This means separating the locs at the base. Don't let your locs grow wild if you want uniform locs and also groom them regularly.

Grooming

Washing and grooming hair biweekly is recommended to "tame" the locs. Even though the locs are not completely established yet, they can handle a little more. Washing carefully is still recommended in this stage. Re-twist and pop after each shampoo. If hair is long enough, locs can be palm rolled to smooth locs. It is crucial to separate locs in this growing stage. If hair is not separated on time, locs will lock together. It will be difficult and painful to separate locs when hair that belongs to one loc is already locked into a neighboring loc. Hair has then to be separated at the scalp, which is not a pleasant experience. Therefore, popping locs can be done more often; perhaps on a weekly basis. If you catch crawling locs, just separate them immediately.

Mature locs

When locs reach maturity after 12 to 18 months, the hair is easy to manage, almost carefree. In this stage you probably have developed a regimen that works for you because hair can be washed and conditioned as often as one pleases and locs can be re-twisted anywhere between biweekly or monthly. It will all depend on the speed of your hair growth and your personal preference. Locs can grow long and can even get too heavy sometimes. If that's the case, go see a loctition to trim your locs or do this yourself because they may break if they get too heavy.

Loc maintenance

There are more ways to groom new growth than palm rolling and re-twisting. A very popular way is the latch hook method. Some prefer this method over palm rolling or re-twisting because once you tighten a loc, the new growth is weaved into the loc. There are no hassles with stray hairs or unraveling of recently twisted new growth. Your hair doesn't have to be wet either. So, in fact, it requires less maintenance.

Be aware of the fact that the way you groom and tighten your locs will be noticeable in the shape of the loc. If you start with re-twisting and change to latching your locs, the part that you latched will be tighter than the part that you twisted. The diameter of your locs will be smaller where you latched and wider where you twisted. People who want to have thinner, tighter locs often use the latch hook method to tighten their locs.

This is how you latch hook your locs:

Figure 20. Latch hook method to tighten locs

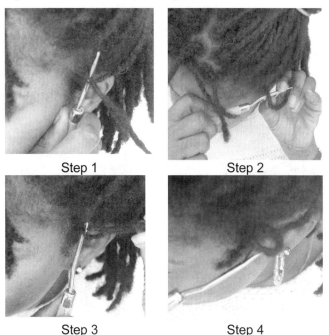

| Step 1 | Step 2 |
| Step 3 | Step 4 |

1. Insert the closed hook into the new growth of a loc. and push it all the way through until the little latch is out past the other side of your hair.

2. Lay your loc on top of the latch hook and close the hook.

3. Gently pull the latch along with your loc back out of the new growth.

4. Remove your loc from the hook.

5. Insert the latch in a different spot in the same loc base, and repeat step one to three, until the new growth is tightened into the loc. You can insert the latch left or right of the original spot or sideways, as long as it is not the same spot. Latching on the same spot will create a hole in your loc. Depending on the amount of new growth it will take three to four runs to tighten a loc.

Finger latching

Finger latching is the same procedure as the latch hook method but without using the tool. You can just use your fingers to push and pull a loc through the base of its new growth to tighten your locs. Like the latch hook method, you should choose a different spot in the base every time you repeat the step.

Push finger through   Pull loc through

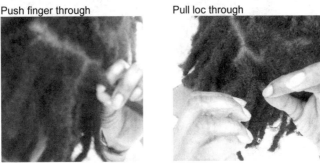

Figure 21. Finger latching

Finger latching is handy if your locs are bigger and don't fit into the latch hook.

If you think about switching from twisting to latching, try it initially on a few locs. If you want uniform locs, stick with one regimen. Locs started with two-strand twists or braids can be latched from the start. Locs started with coils are very likely to unravel in the early stages so latching is hardly possible.

Thread wrapping

Thread wrapping is another way to tame new growth. New growth, broken and stray hairs are wrapped with yarn thread around the base of a loc. This method is also used for thinning locs to strengthen the base of a loc.

Joining locs

When locs are thinning or they grew together at the roots, you can join locs together. You can do this by twisting two locs together and securing them with beads, other jewelry or a thread that matches the color of your locs. If you are joining locs because of thinning, make sure you join a thinning loc to a loc with a stronger base.

Taking down your locs

For many people, cultivating dreadlocks is a holistic experience. Although this does not go for everybody who wears locs, it is without question that locs do have an impact on the person who grows them. Learning to love your hair doing its own thing in its natural state, is a journey that teaches you about yourself, self-love and self-acceptance. Still it is possible that somewhere along the journey one longs for a different hairstyle. There is no harm in wanting another hairstyle after cherishing locs for years. However, growing locs is lot of work so it hurts to shave off luscious locs that have been cherished and cared for for so long. There is an alternative. Instead of shaving off your hair, you can loosen your locs. It is a tedious, hideous job but there is a lot of healthy hair contained in locs. So if you do the job right, you will be rewarded with some good old and fresh naps. Be aware that it will take time to untangle dreadlocks and that you will need a lot of patience. Spread the job over a couple of weeks or even months, depending on the length and the thickness of your locs.

Requirements
Conditioner
Coconut oil
Knitting needle
Wide tooted comb

~ Start with a deep conditioning treatment to soften your locs. Squeeze the conditioner through the locs to completely soften them.

~ Add coconut oil to your locs while the hair is still damp and cover with a hot towel for about five to ten minutes.

~ Cut off the end of the loc so that you have a little puff to start unlocking.

~ Use your fingers to further unravel the loc.

~ If you get stuck, push the knitting needle into the stuck part and pull it down to loosen the part. Then use your fingers again to continue to unravel.

~ When a section is completely unlocked, add conditioner and water, comb through the hair then make a twist or a braid so it blends in with the rest of the locs.

~ Repeat the steps until your hair is completely unlocked.

The golden rules to growing healthy locs

It takes time for hair to grow, so it will also take time to grow long and healthy locs. You will definitely need patience during the early stages but in the end, the reward is priceless: unique and luscious locs will be part of your new personality. If you decide to grow locs, these golden rules may help you beautifully grow them.

1. Do not use beeswax, grease or butters to start your locs.
   Greasy applications will only attract dirt that will make your locs look dull.
2. Less is more: less manipulation and fewer products.
   Do not over twist your locs; leave your hair alone so that locs can settle and do not use conditioners until the hair is fully loced. Slippery agents will keep your strands from locing.
3. Water is your locs' best friend.
   Use water to moisturize and groom your locs and steam to give them body.
4. Natural hair, natural care
   Use herbal rinses to clarify and soften the locs.
5. Get rid of lint immediately before it gets a chance to lock into your hair.
6. Cover your locs at night with a silk or satin scarf to keep them neat.
7. Always twist or palm roll in the same direction, preferably the direction that your hair grows
8. Take the opportunity to learn from each stage and be patient.
9. Enjoy your locs!

Extensions and weaves

There is nothing like natural hair, but if your hair needs a break or time to recover either one, extensions or weaves are a good choice. Whether your hair needs recovery from former abuse or from a hairstyle gone wrong, these methods will stimulate hair growth if the job is done well. You don't have to wear your hair in a style that you are not comfortable with after a hair disaster. A good weave will add length and fullness to one's hair while protecting it. The same goes for extensions that are correctly braided in one's hair. The emphasis should be placed on protecting one's hair. As mentioned before, Afrikan hair grows best if left alone. If your hair is well-protected by extensions or a weave, the hair has a chance to grow undisturbed, free from pulling and environmental threats like the sun. The advantage of weaves and extensions is really is that you can wear any hairstyle while growing your own hair.

Artificial hair types

There are so many types of hair extensions available today that the choices are overwhelming and confusing. So, be prepared before you go shopping for your extensions. Make sure you have a hairstyle in mind and educate yourself on the pros and the cons before you make a choice. Also, be aware of the fact that most artificial hair, even 100 percent human hair, is treated with chemicals. If you are allergic to synthetics or certain chemicals, you might want to test the extensions before you buy and certainly before you attach them to your hair.

Hair Fibers	
PP	Plain Synthetic
KN	Kanekalon
TOYO	Toyokalon

Table 3 Artificial hair fibers

The most popular and common types of artificial hair are basically made of three different synthetic fibers. They are Synthetic, Kanekalon and Tokyokalon.

Acryl Yarn and Lain Yarn
Pros: durable, lightweight

Cons: limited color choice - only black and brown
This type of yarn is light and soft with a matte finish. It is not only durable but also easy to wash and dry. These extensions don't reflect light, which is why they are popular for natural braid and loc styles. Very often, hairstyles with acryl will look better the longer they last. Although this is an advantage, keep in mind that extension styles should not be kept longer than three months.

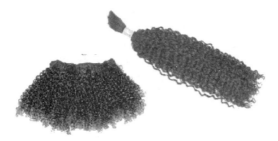

Figure 22. Weave hair: has a track - Bulk hair: loose strands

Linen and Lain yarn
Pros: soft
Cons: Very porous, takes a long time to dry
Unless you don't have a problem not wetting your hair until the style lasts or unless you don't have a problem with hair getting heavy and taking hours to dry, always choose acryl yarn. Yarn is often used for wrapped and braid styles and linen for Senegalese twists and Corkscrew styles. Linen and some types of yarn can get uncomfortably heavy when wet. Ask for advice before you choose these materials. Sometimes a style with these materials should not be washed.

Hair types	Characteristics	Usage
Silky	Thin threads, shiny, flexible	Micro braids, lace braids, invisible braids
Yaky	Course, to resemble straightened hair	Box braids
Afro Kinky	Very light voluminous and Kinky	Senegalese twists, dreadlocks, lace braids

Jumbo	Thin threads, matte, flexible	Braids, cornrows
Bush Baby, Kinky Curly	Medium threads, shiny	Afros, Puffs and combination styles like Cornrows with puffs

Table 4 Table of synthetic hair types

Synthetic

Pros: tremendous variety, inexpensive

Cons: difference in quality

Plain synthetic, PP fiber, or premium acrylic all refer to synthetic fibers. The quality of plain synthetic varies enormously, from less expensive and less durable, to more expensive and more durable. The advantage is the versatility. Almost any type of curl or hairstyle that you can imagine can be imitated with synthetic fiber. Be careful though, some types of really cheap synthetic can literarily cut through natural hair.

Kanekalon

Pros: durable, smooth and soft

Cons: does not expand with natural hair, limited choice (Limited choice of what?)

Kanekalon is a synthetic fiber of good quality. It is usually more expensive than plain synthetic hair but it is also softer and smoother on one's natural hair. The texture, its softness and the fact that it is durable, make this fiber ideal for all kinds of braids and hairstyles. The only disadvantage is that it does not expand as natural hair does when it gets wet. This may increase the tension of the extension on one's hair.

Toyokalon

Pros: durable, smooth and soft

Cons: does not expand with natural hair, limited choice (Again, limited color choices? Explain)

Toyokalon is very much like Kanekalon, it's an advanced version of Kanekalon. Like Kanekalon, it is lighter than synthetic hair and can be used with curling irons (low settings). It is probably the closest resemblance of all synthetics to human hair. That is why it is also the most expensive synthetic type of hair.

Some extensions and many weaves are made from real hair. This could be either human or animal hair.

Yaky

Pros: strong, coarse
Cons: less flexible, tangles easier than human hair
Yaky hair originally comes from the Yak, a domestic Ox from Central Asia. It is thick, coarse hair and is used to resemble Afrikan hair that has been chemically straightened. It is usually referred to as Kinky-Straight hair. Yaky hair is often blended with human hair and sold as 100 percent human hair, for instance as in Human Yaky.

Human hair
Pros: Choice
Cons: easily slips
Collected from different parts of the world, human hair comes in a myriad of textures and colors and is the most expensive type of hair. There is also a tremendous difference in quality depending on how and where the hair was collected and processed. Hair gathered from combing usually delivers lower quality than hair cut from the head. Low-quality hair easily mats and becomes stiff after washing. To check quality, feel if the hair feels soft and if you can easily run your fingers through it. Before using it on your head, see how the hair holds after it gets wet. It is hard to spend valuable time and money only to find your hair a matt filled mess after your first wash.

Extensions

We speak of extensions when imitation hair is integrated into a braiding style. Extensions add length and fullness to one's natural hair and they could be integrated in any kind of hairstyle like cornrows, silky twists or box braids. The most popular box braids are a good example of extensions. We see them everywhere in different lengths, colors and designs. There are a couple of other ways to extend hair today but braiding still is the best for Afrikan hair. None of the techniques that require any kind of heat or glue to attach extensions is recommended for natural hair. Glue or any kind of adhesive damage natural hair when the extensions are removed.

Getting extensions

Once you have decided on a certain hairstyle and you have made your choice in extensions, finding a skilled braider is the next step. This is a most important step. There are many braiders today, but not all of them care about natural hair. They don't know how to handle this type of hair naturally so they will pull your precious naps out of your scalp or even recommend a texturizer to "soften" your kinks. Do not go for any of this if you want to keep your hair. Texturizers are the same as relaxers and adding extensions to hair that has just been chemically treated has disastrous consequences. After a relaxer or texturizer, hair is too weak to hold extensions and your hair will either break off or fall out. A little research can prevent you from these kinds of disasters. If you see women with good-looking braid styles, ask them where they had them done and if they would recommend their salons. Always ask questions. Ask the braider if she knows how to handle natural hair and talk to her about your desired style. Ask about the pros and cons of the extension style regarding your lifestyle. For instance, considering that you work out frequently or that you want to go on a holiday wearing the style. Make sure that the braider also cares about promoting healthy hair more than just collecting the money. Before you get your hair braided, it is also helpful to know the dos and the don'ts of hair braiding.

The do's and the don'ts of hair braiding

~ *Do not keep braids that are too tight*
Regardless if you add extensions or not, excessively tight braids can ruin your hair. They can literally pull hair out causing damage to the hair and scalp. Tight braids can leave bald spots if they damage the hair follicles because hair can't come out if the roots are damaged. So be very careful and take braids out if they are too tight. You know that they are too tight when they give you a headache or you can hardly smile.

~ *Do not wear micros*
Tiny micro braids are fragile and prone to break. Extensions are too heavy for small sections of hair and add stress on the strands. The residue that piles up over time will only worsen this condition and the strands are more likely to break when you take them out.

~ Do not use deep conditioners
Deep conditioners are very hard to wash out when you wear extensions and leave residue behind that builds up. Buildup that gathers around the base of a braid can smother the braid leaving the braids less flexible and add stress on a certain point of the braids. If you wear extensions, avoid products that leave residue.

~ *Do hot oil treatments*
Instead of deep conditioners, do hot-oil treatments to boost the hair. A hot-oil treatment also softens the new growth and the braids without causing buildup. Natural liquid oils are best to use because they penetrate the braids and prevent the scalp from dryness.

~ *Do a touchup*
If you want to keep your hairstyle for two to three months, have a re-braid touchup around the hairline after no more than six weeks. The hairline is most fragile and too much buildup can easily cause these vulnerable, little hairs to break.

~ *Do not keep extensions longer than three months*
The longer you leave extensions in the harder it will be to take them out. Three months is really the maximum period of time that extensions are allowed in hair. After this time, taking extensions out becomes a tedious job because the hair will locs together with the extension.

~ *Do not add extensions while the hair is still wet*
Do not do this especially with cornrows. Think about what happens if you twist your natural hair when it's still wet. When the twists dry, they noticeably shrink a lot, don't they? That is because wet hair is more pliable and stretches more, and kinks naturally shrink when they dry. If you attach extensions to wet hair they will keep your hair from shrinking naturally when your hair dries. This will put extra stress on your scalp and will aggravate the feeling of too-tight braiding. It's worse on cornrows because they are braided on the scalp and that can hurt.

Extension care

Extensions are a rather carefree style, but that doesn't mean that you have to be careless. Some styles like silky twists can't endure water but they also need to be cared for. Every hairstyle needs care.
Always keep the scalp clean as described in Chapter 3 if your style can't endure water and use a natural homemade spray like the Rosemary spray to keep the hair and style fresh. This technique can also be used for cornrows styles if you want to keep them fresh for a longer time.

Extension styles that are able to endure water can be washed the usual way. You can use shampoo on your extensions because your natural hair is protected by the extensions.
To wash:

- wet hair
- apply conditioner/diluted shampoo to your braids
- massage your scalp with the balls your finger to loosen dirt
- wash the braids by starting at the base of the braid and moving down the braid in one direction
- thoroughly rinse the braids by squeezing them in a downward motion without pulling the hair
- rinse with baking soda or ACV rinse to remove traces of shampoo or conditioner in order to prevent buildup
- if you wear cornrows, massage the scalp carefully in between the rows in the direction that the braids flow. If the style becomes frizzy carefully use a soft toothbrush to restyle them. Then tie a scarf and leave it on until the braids are dry.
- Oil the scalp as needed.

Taking extensions out

Sooner or later it will be time to remove the extensions. This is quite a job that requires patience because hair has not been combed for a while and it is very likely that there is buildup at the base of the braids from products, pollution and dust. A hot oil treatment is ideal to loosen the buildup and lubricate the hair at the same time.
Take time to remove extensions. Ask a friend to help you or rent some DVDs but make sure time is on your side because you must not rush this task. It will cost you your hair. Structurally taking the extensions out can make the job a lot easier.

How to structurally take out extensions

- Divide the extensions in six to 12 parts, twirl each part and clip it up.
- Start with one section and cut the extensions an inch from your own hair so that the ends are opening up.
- Start taking the extensions out by loosening each braid individually. Start at the end of the braid and work up to the scalp.
- Once the extension is out, remove all braid debris and untangle.

- Repeat until a whole section is completed. Make a twist of the section and repeat until the head is completed

*Tip: Coconut oil can help loosen dirt and moisturize the strands so that buildup will come out of the hair more easily.

Weaves

For the classic weave, a person's hair is cornrowed along the scalp as a base to attach commercial hair. Usually the cornrow base itself is also done with extensions to create a more supportive base and to protect one's hair. If the base is secure and the person's hair is well protected weft tracks are sewn into the base.

Since the cornrows are the base of the weave, special attention is required. Not only is it important that the cornrow base lies as flat on the scalp as possible so that the hair falls naturally. It is also important that the cornrow pattern matches the desired hairstyle and complements the shape of the head at the same time. A cornrow base that meets the important criteria creates a most natural weave.

The drawback of this method is lumpy tracks. The weft tracks on top of the cornrows can easily make the hair look lumpy, no matter how flat and close to the scalp the cornrows are braided.

The Interlock method creates a more natural look because there are no weft tracks involved. Instead of weft tracks, small portions of loose hair are attached directly to the cornrow base. The result is a more natural hairstyle because of the natural lift and volume. This technique cannot be used for straight hairstyles because straight hair lays flat and may not be able to fully cover the cornrows.

The drawback of this method is that a style does not last longer than eight weeks because the bulk hair easily sheds.

There are several other varieties of weaves and extensions today. In the bonding method, the weft tracks are directly applied to the scalp close to the roots. Although this method is less lumpy, it involves the use of glue. Fusion, bonding and all the other methods that require some kind of glue, latex or surgical type adhesive to attach the hair extensions, are not recommended for the same reasons as mentioned in the paragraph of extensions; using glue damages the hair when the extensions are removed.

Getting a weave

Think about your motives before you choose to weave your hair. The reason you want a weave could be the decisive factor for style. A weave just to grow out a perm is different from a weave that needs to help recover damaged hair or cover up a bold spot. Once you think your motives through, arrange a consultation with a professional stylist to determine the health of your hair and to decide on your styling options.

Like extensions, a competent professional is critical for a good weave style. Make sure that the stylist is a good one who cares for your hair.

The hairline

Naturally concealing the hairline is the most challenging aspect of weaving hair. Hair in the front is most delicate and you should decide whether to incorporate the hairline in the cornrow base or not. Both can be a problem. An obvious weave is a bad one so the cornrow base should not be visible, especially not in the front. An easy solution is wearing a headband or a scarf to conceal this but also ask the hairstylist about her technique's to conceal the hairline. With the natural weave styles, one or two inches around the hairline are left out to naturally mix with the weft hair. The weakness of this solution is that the hair that is out to mix with the artificial hair doesn't grow as much as the part that is weaved. The longer timeframe one wears a weave, the bigger the difference in hair length. Take this into consideration when you decide on a weave.

Caring for weaves

Caring for weaves is rather easy because your own hair should be safely protected so you cannot harm it. The hairstyle and the type of fiber you choose will determine your weave care but usually the emphasis will be on keeping the weft hair from tangling. Combing or brushing is not recommended for weaves because this causes the weft hair to shed from the weave tracks. Use your fingers to untangle to prevent the weave from shedding. If you need to comb or brush, keep one hand on your head while doing so. This will not only prevent too much hair from coming out, it will also prevent disturbing the underlying cornrows.

The do's and the don'ts for weaves

~ *Follow your stylist's advice*
Follow the advice of your stylist regarding how to care for your style; ask how often to wash or condition and if or how often a touch up will be required.

~ *Keep your scalp clean*
This is even more essential for weave styles because the scalp is covered all the time creating a hotbed for bacteria.

~ *Do not sleep on your weave while it is wet or damp*
Do not sleep on your weave if it is still wet or damp. This avoids matting as well as damage to your natural hair. For longer length weaves, tie up the hair before sleeping on it.

~ *Prevent matting*
Remove all tangles before wetting or shampooing hair to prevent irreversible matting.

~ *Do use a scarf*
Sleeping in a cap or scarf will protect your style which will keep it neat for a longer period of time.

~ *Do not keep a weave style in too long*
Three months is the maximum for weaves as well as for extensions. If the cornrows start to mat you risk scalp problems and hair breakage.

~ *Less is more*
Use products sparingly because product residue will build up in the underlying cornrows. If you must use a conditioner or a moisturizer, just use it on the weave. Also rinse thoroughly after washing.

Taking out a weave

Taking out a weave is not as time consuming as removing braid extensions but you have to be careful not to damage your own hair. Ask your stylist where the starting point is and the best way to remove the extensions. If you are handy, you may be able to do this yourself. First, you have to remove the weft hair and then take down the cornrow base. The difficult part is removing the artificial hair.

Appendix A - Hair Structure

Hair is an appendage of the skin and the primary biological function of the strands on our head is to protect our scalp from extreme weather conditions to head injury. The derived function of hair may be to adorn oneself to flaunt and attract the opposite sex as peacocks do in the animal kingdom. Taking a closer look at the structure of hair will certainly serve our interests in growing and keeping beautiful, healthy hair.

Hair is composed of the same kind of material that makes up our finger and toe nails. It is much thinner and it is called keratin. Each strand of hair consists of three layers: the cuticle, the cortex and the medulla. All of the layers are critical to having healthy hair.

The cuticle
The cuticle is composed of several layers of scales overlapping each other. Unlike straight hair where the scales overlap each other like tiles on a roof, the scales of virgin Afrikan hair pile upon each other like plastic cups if they are stacked together. Consequently, kinky hair has up to 12 to 14 layers more than straight hair.
This outermost layer of a hair shaft and responsible for how your hair feels and looks. If this layer is in good shape, your hair feels smooth because the cuticle protects and seals the hair shaft. When the scales are open, your hair will feel rough and will tangle easy because hair shafts with open scales have the tendency to cling to each other.

The cortex
The cortex is middle layer of a hair shaft that determines the color, texture, strength, elasticity and the moisture level in hair. If this layer is in good shape, your hair will be bouncing with tensile strength. On the other hand, if your hair snaps while you try to stretch it, the cortex is probably in bad shape.
The natural pigment called melanin that is present in the cortex is responsible for the color of our hair. And the number and the strength of the sulfur bonds in this layer determine the texture of the hair.

The medulla
The medulla is the deepest layer of a hair shaft and unlike straight hair, the medulla of Afrikan hair is not empty. On the contrary, Afrikan hair has a very strong and pronounced medulla. It contains almost the same components as the cortex except for the melanin and the strength of the

bonds in this layer determine the size of our coils. The stronger the bonds, the tinier the coils.

Hair follicle
Hair emerges out of follicles that are embedded in the scalp. The hair root receives its nutrition from the hair follicle that is connected to the nervous system of the body. Hair prospers by the growth activity in the follicles and good blood circulation.
The number of follicles determines the density of our hair; the more follicles, the denser our hair.
The hair follicle also produces Sebum via the Sebaceous Glands that are attached to it. Sebum is the natural grease that our hair produces to keep hair moisturized and supple. Like perspiration, Sebum is colorless, odorless and sterile. Afrikan hair produces more Sebum than any other hair type and the strong sulfur bonds in the cortex and the medulla, accountable for the kinks, absorb more sebum than any other hair type.
Not all follicles have the same shape. The shape of a hair follicle differs per hair type and varies from oval to round. Afrikan hair has an oval shaped follicle while straight hair has a round-shaped follicle.

Hair growth
Hair grows continuously at an average rate of half an inch a month. The length of time that hair grows depends on the length of time of the growth activity in the follicles. This varies from one to five years. Hair can often grow for a longer period of time but it is exceptional for hair to grow more than eight years at the time.

Hair growth cycle
We speak of the hair growth cycle because hair grows in cycles. After years of growing, a hair strand rests and falls out only to start growing again. The different phases of the hair growth cycle are: the growing phase, the resting phase and the shedding phase.

The growing phase – determines the length of the hair. The longer the growing phase can last, the longer the hair can grow.

Resting phase - after growing several years in a row, hair growth decreases and eventually stops.

Shedding phase – hair roots release the follicle when a new hair emerges. In fact, the new hair pushes out the old one.

Hair grows steadily but not synchronously. Normally about 90 percent of our hair is in the growing phase while the rest of the hair is either in the resting or shedding phase. Hair that naturally comes out while unbraiding or washing is shed hair. You will notice many shedded hairs after wearing extensions for months. Since the hair strands did not have a chance to shed naturally, they stay in the braid until the braid is taken out. Locs are the only hairstyle that does not allow hair to shed. With locs, shedded hair will lock together with hair that is still growing. That is why locs will naturally grow thicker.

Appendix B, How relaxers work

BASED ON RESEARCH BY DR. EDWARD TONY LLONEAU

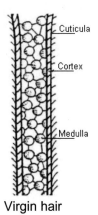

Virgin hair

Magnified view of the cross section of a virgin Afrikan hair shaft. Although a relaxer destroys up to 50% of the cuticle, the alteration of the medulla is what really causes the kinks to break leaving the hair straight. That is why the emphasis here is on the medulla.

 sulfite bonds
(cell structure)

cystien links
connecting the bonds

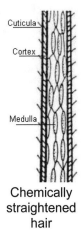

Chemically straightened hair

Figure 23 Hair structure

The process
When a relaxer is applied to the hair, it must penetrate the cuticle, or the outer layer of a hair shaft. To penetrate the hair, relaxers using Sodium Hydroxide as their active ingredient will destroy ½ to ¼ from the hair shaft. As the relaxer is worked into the hair, it scrapes away as much as 1/3 of the cuticle scales. The relaxer next penetrates the Cortex and may lift some natural color. This is why the hair is colored after relaxing the hair.

The next area of the hair shaft affected by the relaxer is the Medulla. As the relaxer is worked into the hair, the hair shaft is stretched by removing a large degree of its elasticity and squeezing out 25 percent of the natural oils.
Cystien links that connect the bonds are changed from their crisscross, up-down, every which way configuration and reformed into a straight up-and-down pattern, reconnecting
the reformed bonds in that manner. (See diagram)

The changing of the cystien links is the main factor for hair being permanent straight as a result of the relaxer treatment. This is also the reason we cannot reconstruct relaxed hair; changing cystien links is irreversible.

After the process:
1. The hair is longer.
2. The hair is thinner.
3. Up to 50 percent of the cuticle is gone.
4. Sulfur bonds are elongated instead of round.
5. Cystien links now connect the bond in a straight configuration instead of a cross manner.
6. Some color has been lifted from the cortex.
7. Up to ½ of the natural oils contained in the bonds have been removed.

Glossary

ACV Rinse: Apple Cider Vinegar rinse. A finishing rinse of apple cider vinegar that clarifies neutralizes and promotes detangling after washing the hair.

Afro Puff: Afrikan hair pulled back together with an afro-like end

Alopecia: Medical term for hair loss or baldness in general.

BAA: A very big afro.

Banding: A hairstyle that is used as a technique to stretch the hair naturally without using damaging heat.

Big Chop: Cutting the processed part of the hair strands off leaving one's natural hair.

Box braids: Loose hanging braids with or without extensions.

Braid locs: Cultivated locs originated by braids.

Braids: Three strands of sectioned hair twisted around each another.

Buildup: Product residue that leaves a film over the strands and stiffens the hair.

Casama Braids: Large, single braids with a tight stitch that are tapered and/or curved at the ends.

Clarifying treatment: A treatment to get rid of buildup and residue.

Conditioner Wash: See "No-Poo"

Cornrows: Three-strand braids interwoven to lay flat on the scalp

Comedogenic: Ingredients that clog pores and may cause acne.

Creamy Crack: Addiction to relaxers.

Curl Definition: A tight kink form without frizz.

Cuticle: The outermost layer of the hair.

Dandruff: Hair condition that causes the scalp to flake.

Deep Conditioner: A formula designed to improve the health of one's hair.

Dreadlocks: Meshed hair that has grown and loced together.

Earth locs: See dreadlocks.

Emollients: Supple, lubricating or thickening agents that prevent water loss and have a softening and soothing effect on hair.

Emulisifier: An agent used to mix two non-mixable liquids like water and oil into a homogenized emulsion.

Fine Hair: Hair that has thin hair strands.

Finger-comb: Untangling and styling hair with fingers instead of using a comb or a pick.

Finger-parting: Sectioning hair with fingers instead of with a comb or a pick.

Flat Twist: One or two-sectioned braid flatly interlocked on the scalp.

Follicles: The pores in the skin from which hair strands emerge and grow.

Free form locs: locs that naturally develop after one stops to comb hair.

'Fro: Abbreviation for afro.

Geni-locs: Yarn wrapped around single brands to resemble locs.

Hand In 'Fro Disease (HIFD): A person who is unable to keep her hands out of her hair.

Humectant: Water-binding agent or water-attracting agents that help hair strands to retain water (moisture).

Keratin: The type of protein and the major constituent of the outer layer of the skin, nails, and hair.

Leave-in Conditioner: A hair product to soften hair and doesn't need to be rinsed out.

Locs or locs: See dreadlocks.

Loctitian: Hair dresser specialized in grooming locs.

LOL: Means Laughing Out Loud. An abbreviation that is used very often on the World Wide Web in chat rooms, emails and forums.

Lo-Poo: No-poo but still using shampoo occasionally

Medulla: Inner layer of a hair shaft

Melanin: Pigment that gives hair its natural color.

Molding Crème: A rather thick substance to enhance and shape curls.

Napptural: From the website napptruality.com. It means naturally nappy hair.

No Poo: An abbreviation for no shampoo and the same thing as conditioning wash. It means washing your hair with an instant conditioner instead of a shampoo. This idea comes from the book Curly Girl where writer Lorraine Massey explains that she stopped using shampoo. She never uses shampoo anymore and her hair looks and feels so much better because shampoo strips curly hair of natural moisture. Although the writer has curly hair, many of us with Afrikan hair adopted the idea after it was posted on Nappturality.com. It soon became normal in this community because it made a world of difference.

Organic locs: See free-form locs.

Panthenol: Also referred to as Pro-Vitamin B5 used as a nourishing, conditioning agent in hair aids.

Papilla: The root of a hair shaft that connects the hair to the nerve systems of the body in order to nourish the hair.

pH: Stands for "potential of hydrogen." Provides a measure on a scale from zero to 14 of the acidity or alkalinity of a solution; seven is neutral, greater than seven is acidic and less than seven is basic.

Plopping: A styling technique to wear afro hair out.

Pomade: A very rich and thick hair aid used to tame frizz, provide hold or slick back hair completely.

Product Junkie: A person addicted to hair products.

Protective Hairstyles: Hairstyles that don't expose the ends of the hair in order to protect them.

Puff: See "afro puff."

Revitalizer: An intensive conditioner to strengthen damaged hair.

Scab Hair: Hair that comes out after it has been affected by chemicals. It feels unnaturally hard and crunchy.

Sebum: The oil that hair roots naturally produce to lubricate hair

Spicy locs: Locs that are "spiced up" with little pieces of extensions attached to the ends to add color or give locs a unique look.

Shrinkage: Kinky and curly hair is always longer if you stretch it. Shrinkage is the difference between the actual length and to length the hair appears to be.

Silky Twist: Rolled and gelled flat twists.

Sisterlocks: Cultivated locs.

Split Ends: Ends of hair strands that are damaged.

Styling Gel: A light solution to ease frizz and add shine.

Surfactant: Acronym for surface active agent. A substance used to emulsify oils and keep dirt in suspension so that it can be rinsed away with water.

Texturizer: A relaxer that is applied on the hair for a very short time. Hair goes through the exact same process as when the hair is relaxed and the process can be as harmful as such a treatment.

Transitioners: Women who are in the process of transferring from chemical processed to natural hair.

Trichology: Hair science; medical study and treatment of hair and scalp.

TWA: Abbreviation for Teeny Weeny Afro.

Volumizer: Styling aid to add body and volume to hair.

Bibliography

Bailey, Diane Carol. Natural Hair Care and Braiding.
Canada: Milady Publishing, 1998.

Kinard Tulani. No Lye.
New York: St Martin's Griffin, 1997.

Ferrell, Pamela. Let's talk hair.
Washington: Cornrows & Co, 1996.

Massey, Lorraine. Curly Girl
New York: Workman Publishing Company, Inc.

Hair in African Art and Culture. The Museum of African Art.
New York: The Museum of African Art, 2000.

Shamboosie. Beautiful black hair: Real Solutions to Real Problems.
Phoenix, Amber books 2202.

Drs Khumalo, P. T. Doe, R. P. R. Dawber and D.J.P Ferguson, phD. What's
normal African hair? A light and scanning electron-microscopic study. From
the Department of Dermatology, the Churchill Hospital & Nuffield
Department of Pathology, John Radcliffe Hospital, Oxford, United Kingdom
2000.

Draelos, ZD. Understanding African-American hair. From the Department of
Dermatology, Bowman Gray School of Medicine, Wake Forest University,
Winston-Salem, NC, USA 1997.

Dr. Edward Tony Lloneau. The complete explanation of hair types and
structure, A brief history of hair relaxing, How chemicals used in
cosmetology services permanently change the hair.

Sisterlocks: Dr. JoAnne Cornwell.

Riqui Locs: Richelle Braithwaite.

Braids through the ages; Essence May, 1998

Photography

Front cover pictures from left to right: Dolores Leeuwin, Riqui by Kevin Duke, Satcha Valies, Mireille Liong, Sharyn Sawyer by M. Liong, Jenteel Pierre by M. Liong, Sandy Weeks by Jeff Liong-A-Kong, Mireille Liong by Harvey Wirht, Nicole Simson by Aart den Hartog, Roshini by M. Liong, Fatima by M. Liong, Mireille Liong by Harvey Wirht, Rachelle by M. Liong, Kaissa Cameroonian singer by Maciek Schejbal, Satcha Valies, Mamke by M. Liong, Roline Deel by Aart den Hartog.

Other pictures:
Figure 8 – Deidre Small. Hair by Deidre.
Figure 11 – Jenteel. Hair by Jenteel.
Figure 14 – Terza Sanches. Hair by Terza.
Figure 16 – Sherize Grep. Hair by Nicole Simson.
Figure 17 – Graciella Perzon. Hair by Norine Abena, hair salon Zusbena.
Figure 18 – Jacqueline Ammah a.k.a Sweet Africa. Hair by Jacqueline.
Figure 19 – Sisterlocks™ picture of Joanne Cornwel
Figure 19 – Spicy locs. Hair by Richelle Braithwaite a.k.a. Riqui.

Footnotes

[1] PBS: Trade Secrets: http://www.pbs.org/tradesecrets, 2001. Download date: 4/5/2004

[2] Rio, a so called natural relaxer was banned after the FDA received the largest number of complaints ever about a cosmetic product; it caused instant hair loss, severe scalp irritations and other scalp and skin conditions.

[3] Aubrey organics: http://www.aubrey-organics.com, http://www.healthy-communications.com/harmfulingredients1.html, http://www.healthy-communications.com/

[4] CIR: Cosmetic Ingredient established by the Cosmetic, Toiletry & Fragrance Association (CTFA) with support of the U.S. Food & Drug Administration (FDA) and the Consumer Federation of America to independently review and assesses the safety of ingredients used in cosmetics industry.

[5] Beauty to die for-Judy Vance

[6] Ethers cause adverse reactions, are known to be toxic and can cause contact dermatitis.

[7] Beauty to die for by Judi Vance, Natural Organic Hair and Skin care by Aubrey Hampton.

[8] Beauty to die for by Judi Vance, Natural Organic Hair and Skin care by Aubrey Hampton.

[9] Beauty to die for by Judi Vance, Natural Organic Hair and Skin care by Aubrey Hampton.

[10] Beauty to die for by Judi Vance, Natural Organic Hair and Skin care by Aubrey Hampton.

[11] Beauty to die for by Judi Vance, Natural Organic Hair and Skin care by Aubrey Hampton.

[12] Beauty to die for by Judi Vance, Natural Organic Hair and Skin care by Aubrey Hampton.

[13] Beauty to die for by Judi Vance, Natural Organic Hair and Skin care by Aubrey Hampton.

[14] (Sources: "Skin Care—From the Inside Out and Outside In," Tufts Daily, April 1, 2002; eMedicine Journal, May 8, 2002, volume 3, number 5, www.emedicine.com; Cutis, February 2001, pages 25–27; and Contact Dermatitis, January 1996, pages 12–16)

[15] Beauty to die for by Judi Vance, Natural Organic Hair and Skin care by Aubrey Hampton.

[16] No poo method or condition wash.

[17] Spicy locs; fully loced hair spiced up with little pieces of extensions at the end of a loc by Richelle Braitwaite.